They stood there for a long, long moment, saying nothing, just holding each other.

Then she tipped her head back.

Whatever she'd been about to say was lost to the London evening, because his eyes were oh, so dark and all the words went out of her head. His mouth was very slightly parted. She could see the beginnings of a beard on his face, and unable to stop herself, she reached up to glide her fingertips across his skin, feeling the catch of stubble.

Daniel sucked in a breath.

And then he twisted his head so his mouth brushed her palm. His lips were warm and soft, and she ached to feel them against hers.

This shouldn't be happening.

But now it had started, she couldn't stop it. Didn't *want* to stop it.

She wasn't sure which of them moved first, but the next thing she knew, her arms were around his neck, his arms had tightened around her waist and he was kissing her, his mouth sweet and gentle, offering temptation as well as comfort.

Dear Reader,

When you've written a lot of romances, it's quite hard to find something fresh—and I really hate the idea of repeating myself and disappointing my readers.
(I admit I have favorite tropes, but I do try to make the conflicts different!)

I wanted to focus on an older couple, nearer my age group, this time around. And I wanted to break a rule or two. My heroine was cheated on by a very charming man. So who's the worst person she could fall for? A charming TV doctor. Worse still, it turns out that he made a mistake and ruined his own marriage half a lifetime ago. His ex forgave him, but he never truly forgave himself.

How do you atone for the past? What happens if you risk giving someone a second chance, but deep down they don't feel they deserve it and can't accept it?

So this book is looking at love from a different angle. Where your boundaries are. How you can change. And how, finally, you can accept yourself for who you are and move on to find happiness.

I hope you enjoy Mandy and Daniel's journey.

With love,

Kate Hardy

PEDIATRICIAN'S UNEXPECTED SECOND CHANCE

KATE HARDY

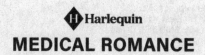

MEDICAL ROMANCE

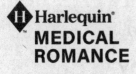

Harlequin®
MEDICAL ROMANCE

Recycling programs for this product may not exist in your area.

ISBN-13: 978-1-335-94278-4

Pediatrician's Unexpected Second Chance

Harlequin Enterprises ULC
22 Adelaide St. West, 41st Floor
Toronto, Ontario M5H 4E3, Canada
www.Harlequin.com

Printed in U.S.A.

Kate Hardy has always loved books and could read before she went to school. She discovered Harlequin books when she was twelve and decided that this was what she wanted to do. When she isn't writing, Kate enjoys reading, cinema, ballroom dancing and the gym. You can contact her via her website, katehardy.com.

Books by Kate Hardy

Harlequin Medical Romance

Twin Docs' Perfect Match

Second Chance with Her Guarded GP
Baby Miracle for the ER Doc

Yorkshire Village Vets

Sparks Fly with the Single Dad

Surgeon's Second Chance in Florence
Saving Christmas for the ER Doc
An English Vet in Paris

Harlequin Romance

Snowbound with the Brooding Billionaire
One Week in Venice with the CEO
Crowning His Secret Princess
Tempted by Her Fake Fiancé
Wedding Deal with Her Rival

Visit the Author Profile page
at Harlequin.com for more titles.

For all the readers who've been on this journey
with me for nearly half a lifetime—
thank you for your support xx

CHAPTER ONE

'MUM? WHAT HAVE you done to your eye?'

Mandy stifled a groan. If her bloodshot eye was visible to her daughter on a small phone screen, then it was going to be *really* obvious in real life. Just what she didn't need on her first day in her new job. 'I'm fine,' she said. 'I must've sneezed in my sleep, or something, and burst a blood vessel in my eye. It'll go away by itself in three or four days. And, no, it doesn't hurt. Stop fussing.'

'I'm nearly seven months pregnant. I'm *allowed* to fuss,' Gemma said with a grin. 'I'm not going to hold you up. I just wanted to wish you good luck on your first day.' Her grin broadened. 'Mind you, if you go in with a pirate's eye patch, it'll fascinate all the kids. The ones who are crying will stop and ask if you're Captain Hook's sister, and the ones who aren't crying will perk up and ask if you've got a ticking crocodile following you. Or perhaps a parrot for your shoulder.' She squawked meaningfully. 'You could always pretty up an eye patch. Stick on some sequins and some lace. Actually, no—that can be my class's task this morning, to design you an eye patch. The prettier, the better.'

'If I turn up wearing an eye patch covered in sequins, then my new job-share's going to think the hospital's hired someone who either won't take the job seriously, or is trying a bit too hard to get featured on his TV show,' Mandy said drily.

'Ah, yes. Dr Sexy.' Gemma laughed. 'Do you know how many of my colleagues have asked me if you'll give him their phone number?'

Daniel Monroe—Mandy's fellow joint Head of Paediatrics—was also the star of *London Victoria Children's Ward*, a documentary that showed life in the Paediatric Department and the sheer bravery of their young patients. He was the epitome of tall, dark—well, with a fair sprinkling of grey in his hair—and handsome. Add twinkling brown eyes behind his glasses, a slight scruffiness to his haircut that made women want to fuss over him, and the kind of smile that made female pulses beat a lot faster, and it was no wonder that most of the press referred to him as 'the thinking woman's crumpet'.

Every single female of Mandy's acquaintance had given an envious sigh when they found out who was going to be her job-share.

Not that she'd actually met him yet, because Daniel had been laid low by a virus the day before she'd gone for her interview so he'd had to drop out of the interview panel. But the senior nurse who'd taken her round the ward afterwards had told her that Daniel was even nicer to work with than he seemed on the TV. Calm, capable and kind. He respected the nursing team, and he gave junior doctors a chance to blossom.

In short, Daniel Monroe was a dream doctor.

And this was a dream job. Mandy would spend two days a week in charge of training, while Daniel headed up the department; two days a week heading up the department, while Daniel filmed his documentary; and the other day working with Daniel on admin and strategy. Though their separate roles would also have a fair amount of crossover.

She shook herself. 'He's probably very happily married.'

'Nope. He's definitely single,' Gemma corrected. 'Angelica at work checked him out on social media. And I'm under instructions that I'm not to go on maternity leave next month without getting at least one person's telephone number to him.'

'Tell them your mother's difficult and you daren't ask her,' Mandy said.

'Too late. They've met you. They already know you're perfect.'

'Perfect?' Mandy couldn't help laughing. 'Thank you for the compliment, darling, but I'm far from that. I'll settle for being OK.'

'You're more than OK, Mum. You're going to be a brilliant head of department.'

'*Joint* head,' Mandy reminded her.

'Still brilliant,' Gemma insisted. 'I'm proud of you. So's Dev—' her husband '—and so's The Bump.'

Her first grandchild. When had she suddenly become old enough to be a grandmother? She still felt as if she were twenty-five. 'I'm proud of you all, too,' Mandy said.

'Have a fabulous first day, Mum. Dev's cooking a special dinner so you can tell us all about it tonight. Spiced paneer tikka with baby spinach, lemon dhal, and parathas.'

'You know I'm only coming for Dev's dhal, and not to see you or the bump,' Mandy said, her face deadpan.

Gemma gave a rich chuckle. 'Dev's dhal is responsible for the bump.'

Which served her right for teasing. 'TMI!' Mandy said, making exaggerated gestures of horror. 'It's supposed to be my generation making yours cringe, you know, not the other way round.'

'Bring it on,' Gemma said, her eyes sparkling. 'Right, your challenge is to date someone. For the first time in about—well, you'd need a whole library of calendars to calculate how many years it's been since *you* last dated someone.' Worry bubbled up from behind her daughter's teasing. 'Mum. I really hate to think of you being lonely.'

'Of course I'm not lonely,' Mandy said. 'I have you, Dev, the bump-to-be, Aunty Jen, Gran and Linda. I have book club on the first Monday of the month, ballet class on Fridays, and dance aerobics on Tuesday and Thursday. I'll be your permanent babysitter on Wednesdays so you and Dev get a date night every week, and I'm just about to start a new job. Between my family, my social life and work, I don't have *time* to be lonely.'

'That's not what I…' Gemma stopped herself and sighed. 'Love you, Mum.'

'Love you, too,' Mandy said. 'I'll see you tonight.'

'We're eating at seven. Come whenever you like. And have a brilliant, brilliant day.'

Wearing glasses instead of contact lenses meant that Mandy could get away without wearing eye make-up, and hopefully the tortoiseshell frames of her narrow glasses hid some of the redness in her right eye. Thankfully her skin wasn't having a bad menopause day, so a tinted moisturiser and a neutral lip colour were enough to make her look professional.

Her mum and her sister Jen both texted.

Good luck on your first day!

Her best friend Linda sent a picture of a cute spaniel puppy with the message:

You'll be pawsome!

And even the weather was on her side; although it was grey and a bit on the chilly side, a typical October London day, it wasn't raining. She caught the Tube from King's Cross to Victoria, and walking briskly to the hospital meant she didn't feel the cold.

Mandy had to check the hospital map in the reception area to remind herself where the children's ward was. Hopefully it wouldn't take too long before these corridors felt as familiar as those of Muswell Hill, the hospital where she'd worked for the last fifteen years, she thought as she headed down the corridor.

Before she had the chance to start feeling nervous, she pressed the intercom button on the wall outside the ward.

'Good morning. How can I help?' a voice crackled through the grille.

'Good morning. It's Amanda Cooke. I'm starting work here today, so I don't have my staff card yet and I need someone to let me in,' she said.

'Great—we're expecting you. I'll buzz you in. I'm Khaj, one of the nurses. You'll see me as soon as you walk in. I'm updating the whiteboard.'

The door buzzed, and Mandy made sure she closed it again behind her without anyone following her in; security in vulnerable wards was important. She glanced over towards the reception desk and saw a cheerful-looking nurse in scrubs writing names on a whiteboard, which showed which team members were looking after the patients in each bay.

'Welcome to the London Victoria, Ms Cooke,' the nurse said with a smile.

Mandy smiled back. 'Nice to meet you, Khaj. And please call me Mandy.'

'Mandy.' Khaj looked concerned. 'What happened to your eye?'

Oh. So her glasses really weren't enough to hide the redness. It looked as if she was going to be explaining this all day, then. 'Subconjunctival haemorrhage. I woke up with it this morning so I must've sneezed in my sleep,' Mandy said ruefully.

'Poor you,' Khaj said sympathetically.

'My daughter said I should wear an eye patch,'

Mandy said. 'I have the nastiest feeling she's going to get her class to design one today. And a five-year-old's idea of an eye patch means I'm definitely going to regret buying that pack of off-cuts in the fabric shop for her class's craft box.'

'You sew? Oh, you're definitely going to go down well here,' Khaj said, looking pleased. 'There's a teenager I need to introduce you to later. Now, let's get you loaded up with coffee before I take you through to Daniel.'

'Thank you.' Mandy indicated the bag she was carrying, containing a plastic tub, a box and a bag of apples. 'I brought goodies to say hello to the team. Can I leave them in the staff kitchen?'

'You most certainly can,' Khaj said. 'By the way, your ID card isn't here yet, but I'll get someone to chase that up for you. In the mean-time, just buzz the intercom when you need to be let back in on the ward.'

'Cheers,' Mandy said.

While Khaj made two mugs of coffee—one of which was bright orange and emblazoned with the words 'Dr TWC', which told Mandy that Daniel's colleagues ribbed him mercilessly about his reputation as the Thinking Woman's Crumpet in the media—Mandy put the tub of home-made brownies on the worktop so any-one who walked into the staff kitchen would see them, along with a couple of packets of individually wrapped gluten-free lemon cakes, and some apples for anyone who didn't eat cake. Hopefully she'd covered all dietary requirements and not left anyone out. She left a note on top of the tub:

Look forward to meeting everyone on the ward. Brownies are egg-free and dairy-free; lemon cakes are GF. Cheers, Mandy

'Do you know if Mr Monroe would prefer brownies or lemon cake?' she asked.

Khaj laughed. 'Daniel likes anything sweet. He really deserves to be thirty pounds heavier than he is. We'd hate him for being able to scoff cake with impunity, except he's one of the good guys.'

Brownies, Mandy decided, and wrapped one in a piece of paper towel. And it was good to have reassurance that her new job-share partner was well liked.

She followed Khaj down the corridor, and the nurse rapped on an open door. 'Good morning, Dan. Here's your first appointment of the day. Don't dump all your filing on her.'

'As if I'd do something so underhand,' Daniel drawled, looking up from his desk.

Daniel Monroe on screen was a heartthrob; Daniel Monroe in the flesh was utterly gorgeous. And Mandy really hoped her face didn't look as red as her eye, because it certainly felt hot enough.

'You must be Amanda Cooke. Lovely to meet you at last.' His eyes narrowed. 'What did you—?'

'—do to my eye?' she finished wryly. 'I woke up with it this morning. It could've been a cough, a sneeze, carrying a heavy bag—anything.'

'Subconjunctival haemorrhage,' he said with a grimace. 'Sorry. You've probably had to explain it to half a dozen people already.'

'Yes, and no doubt I'll have to do it for the rest of the day. Still, it's a way of breaking the ice. Have a home-made brownie,' Mandy said, and gave him the paper towel containing the cake. 'I made them last night to say hello to the department.'

'You brought in home-made cake on your first day? Oh, I like you already,' he said with a grin. 'Welcome to the department. I think she's a keeper, Khaj,' he added in a stage whisper.

'Don't badger her into doing your filing,' Khaj repeated sternly. 'I'll leave you with him, Mandy.'

'Of course I won't expect you to do my filing,' Daniel said, rolling his eyes when Khaj had left. 'Though I admit I need nagging to do it. I'd rather clean up projectile vomit, poonami diarrhoea or a pus-filled wound than… Well.' He indicated his very full in-tray.

'We all have bits of the job we hate,' Mandy said lightly.

'Welcome to the London Victoria. We use first names rather than formality here, so may I call you Amanda?' He stood up and held his hand out.

'Mandy,' she said, taking his hand and shaking it. His handshake was firm and dry, but his smile disconcerted her because it really did make her heart feel as if it had just throbbed. She hadn't felt a pull of attraction like this to someone in years, and she was going to have to get a firm grip on that reaction. He was her new colleague, and—even though she knew he was single—she wasn't looking for any relationship other than a professional one. She'd learned the hard way that charm was usually partnered with unreliability, and she wasn't going to forget it.

Oh, help. Amanda Cooke's handshake was firm and professional, but her skin was warm and soft—and it made Dan feel all quivery. The kind of quiver he hadn't felt towards anyone in a very long time, because he always kept his relationships light and fluffy and very, very short. And that meant not dating anyone he worked with.

This woman could be seriously dangerous to his peace of mind.

He shook himself mentally. Talk about an

inappropriate reaction—and it was bad timing as well.

Focus, he told himself. *She's your new job-share. You've just met her. You don't want her to think you're a total numpty.*

'Everyone calls me Dan,' he said. 'Sorry I didn't meet you at your interview.'

'I completely understand. They told me you'd gone down with a virus,' she said.

'The usual occupational hazard of working in Paediatrics,' he said with a rueful smile. 'I probably could have dosed myself up and dragged myself in, but I didn't want everyone who'd been in the same room as me to feel grim as I did, the next morning.'

'That's considerate,' she said. 'Thank you.'

He looked at her. 'I thought we'd take today to settle you in and plan workloads. I've been muddling along for a while; it's going to be so much better for the team having you here. Obviously the ward needs one of us in charge while the other one's teaching or filming, and we need a day together to make sure we iron out any issues that crop up and deal with the suits, plus share the on-call rota at weekends. I normally film on Thursday and Friday when we're working on a series—the new one starts next week—but we can move things round if that doesn't work with your teaching commitments. And I thought we could alternate weekends on call; we can always swap if one of us has something special on.'

She looked surprised, as if she'd expected him to dictate the schedule to her. 'That all works fine for me,' she said.

'Good. And please don't feel awkward about the TV stuff. If you've got an interesting case, I'd be delighted to look at including it on the show; but if you'd rather avoid the cameras completely, that's also fine.' He indicated the orange mug with a sigh. 'As you can see, the team won't let me get away with trying to be a luvvie. That was last year's Secret Santa present. I still can't work out who got it for me; I think they were all in cahoots because they all *really* enjoyed watching me open it.' He grinned. 'But I'll forgive them for teasing, because they also filled it with caramel chocolates.'

'Chocolate's the way to your heart? I'll remember that.'

Daniel really hoped that he didn't look as red and flustered as he felt. Because the glint in her lovely brown eyes made him imagine lying against a pillow while she fed him squares of caramel-filled chocolate, teasing him by rubbing it along his lower lip and then holding it just out of reach and demanding a kiss before she handed over the chocolate…

Oh, for pity's sake. He was fifty-five, not fifteen. Fantasies like that shouldn't be filling his head, particularly in work hours. Despite her red eye, Mandy looked completely cool, calm and professional: which was what he needed to be, too. Preferably right now.

'Let me introduce you to the team,' he said. 'Then we'll grab something to drink—the canteen here does decent coffee—and we can talk about your teaching, training plans for the staff here, and work out our schedules.'

'Sounds good to me,' she said.

Daniel was as good as his word, introducing Mandy to the whole team—from the most junior health care assistant up to the senior consultants. Not only was he on first-name terms with everyone, it was clear from the way he talked that he actually knew all the staff and what mattered to them. They all seemed to bloom in his presence. The patients, too, all had a smile for Dr Dan, whether they were an out-of-sorts toddler or a grumpy teenager.

Perhaps she'd been unfair to him, assuming that his charm meant he was like all the other charming but shallow men she'd met; maybe there really was depth underneath Daniel's surface allure.

Finally, they went into the Paediatric Intensive Care Unit.

'Mo, this is Amanda Cooke, who's sharing the Head of Department role with me,' he said, introducing her to the consultant on the unit. 'Mandy, this is Mohammed Singh, our paediatric intensive care specialist.'

'Nice to meet you—and please call me Mandy,' she said, shaking Mo's hand. 'I'd like to have a meeting with you at some point in the week to discuss training, whenever works for you, to talk about the new intake of students at the university and what we can offer them here. Plus I'd like to know what your team's needs are so I can make sure they're covered.'

'That sounds good,' he said. 'Nice to meet you, too, Mandy.' He looked at Daniel. 'I'm glad you're here, Dan, because I've got a potential case for your show. Though it's a tricky one and I haven't got a firm diagnosis at the moment.'

'That's unusual for you. Want to pick our brains?' Daniel asked.

'Definitely,' Mo said. 'I'll give you the background: the Emergency Department sent eight-month-old Noah Carmichael up to us this morning. His parents took him to the walk-in centre yesterday because he seemed lethargic, was a bit constipated and wasn't feeding well. His mum also thought his cry sounded funny and a bit weaker than normal. The GP told them to keep a close eye on him and bring him to the

Emergency Department here if he got any worse. They didn't sleep much last night, worrying about him, and about five o'clock this morning the mum went in to check on him and discovered he was floppy. They rushed him straight here.'

From years of experience, Mandy knew that very young children could become very unwell, very quickly, and a floppy baby usually meant the little one was really poorly. 'Good call,' she said. 'Does he have any other symptoms?'

'That's where it gets weird,' Mo said. 'He's drooling, his eyelids are droopy and his pupils are a bit sluggish. I was thinking it might be some kind of cerebral virus, except he hasn't got even a hint of a fever.'

'So it's unlikely to be one of the usual viruses, then,' Daniel said, frowning.

'There are signs of bulbar palsies,' Mo added. Bulbar palsies were a set of clinical conditions that occurred when the lower cranial nerves were damaged, possibly by a stroke or a tumour. 'There's also moderate hypotonia.'

Muscle weakness, Mandy thought. The baby was constipated, drooling, not feeding, and had droopy eyelids. No fever. Mo was right; it was an odd set of symptoms. With a virus, she would've expected a fever. But something rang a bell in the back of her head.

'We've intubated him and put him in an induced coma while we run some more tests,' Mo said. 'Starting with a CT scan to see if there's anything obvious causing the bulbar palsies. That's where he is at the moment. He's due back on the ward any minute now.'

'Were there any complications with the birth?' Daniel asked.

'No. Labour and birth were both as standard as it gets, and he's been between the fiftieth and sixtieth centile on all the development charts all the way along,' Mo said. 'His parents didn't have a thing to worry about until yesterday.'

'You mentioned hypotonia. Is there any evidence of paralysis, especially if it's symmetrical and heading downwards?' Mandy asked. 'And do his facial features look flattened at all?'

'His face does look a bit flat, yes,' Mo said. 'Paralysis…obviously he's in an induced coma at the moment, but that's a good point.'

'What are you thinking, Mandy?' Daniel asked.

'It's something a friend came across when she did a couple of years on a job-swap in America,' Mandy said. 'It's really rare here in England, but I think we might be talking about infant botulism.'

'That's so rare I've only ever read about it in medical journals,' Daniel said. 'I've never actually seen a case.'

'Me neither,' Mo said. 'And I've been qualified for twenty years.'

'I haven't seen one myself, either,' Mandy said. 'But this sounds really like the case my friend told me about. If someone's given Noah some honey, he might have swallowed *Clostridium botulinum* spores.'

'In an adult or a baby over the age of one, those spores would go through the digestive system too quickly to cause a problem. But Noah's digestive system is still immature, so the spores would've had time to colonise his large intestine and produce botulinum neurotoxin,' Daniel said thoughtfully.

'Which affect the nerve endings—and that would account for the hypotonia and bulbar palsies,' Mandy agreed.

'Given the other differential diagnoses, I'm not sure if that makes me feel more or less worried,' Mo said. 'The Carmichaels seem pretty switched on, the sort who read every parenting book and magazine going. I can't imagine they would've allowed anyone to give their infant son honey, not when all the health visitors and GPs are so clear with the message about not giving honey to babies under the age of one.'

'They might not have been the ones to give it to him. If a well-meaning older friend or relative took the view that they'd had honey as a baby and it hadn't hurt them, so it wouldn't hurt Noah…' Daniel spread his hands. 'Then his parents wouldn't have known anything about it until it was too late.'

'We need to get a stool sample to the lab,' Mandy said. 'And, if I'm right, we'll need to start treating him with antitoxin.' She grimaced. 'The only thing is, because infant botulism is so rare over here, it's unlikely that any of the hospitals in this country has a stock of infant antitoxin. We certainly didn't have any at Muswell Hill.'

'Where's likely to have it?' Mo asked.

'The head of Pharmacy will know—or at least know where to check,' Daniel said.

'Worst-case scenario, we'll have to ask the pharmacy to talk to the public health department in California, and have the antitoxin couriered here and expedited through Customs,' Mandy said. 'What I do know is that it could take a few days to get the lab results back, and we can't wait for them. The quicker we can start the treatment, the quicker Noah will recover.'

'Including from the paralysis?' Mo asked.

'Yes, but it could take a while, depending on how long it takes for his nerve endings to grow again,' Mandy warned. 'Can we talk to his parents?'

'Of course. They're waiting in the relatives'

room while Noah's having his scan,' Mo said. 'I'll introduce you.'

As Mo introduced them to Lucy and Rob Carmichael, Mandy thought Noah's parents both looked worn out with worry, their faces pallid with dark shadows smudged beneath their eyes. And what she was about to tell them was a parent's worst nightmare.

'Hang on—aren't you the doctor off that telly programme?' Rob asked, looking at Daniel.

'Yes, but I'm also a qualified senior doctor who works here, so please don't worry about the TV presenter stuff,' Daniel said. He gave them both a reassuring smile. 'Mo's told us about your son, and you did absolutely the right thing bringing Noah here when you were concerned.'

Rob looked miserable. 'He's so poorly. Dr Singh had to put him in a coma, and nobody seems to know what's making Noah sick.'

'We're running tests to rule some things out, and the CT scan will hopefully give us a better idea of what might be causing Noah's symptoms,' Daniel said gently. 'The three of us have been talking about his symptoms, and my colleague Mandy might have worked out what the problem is.'

'It's a strange question, but is there any chance that someone might have given Noah honey or any kind of preserved food in the last couple of days?' Mandy asked.

'Honey?' Lucy looked shocked. 'Of course not. You're not supposed to give a baby honey because it might make them ill.'

Exactly what Mo had suggested Noah's mum's response would be. But Daniel had also had a suggestion about where the honey might have come from. 'We were wondering, could someone else have given him anything with honey in it? A cookie or a piece of cake, maybe?' Mandy asked. 'Something that somebody made at home, perhaps, or maybe from a toddler group bake sale? And Mo said it was yesterday he started being ill, so maybe he ate something on Friday or Saturday that started affecting him yesterday?'

'He was with us on Saturday,' Lucy said. 'But on Fridays, we both work and my mum has him for the day. She takes him to a baby music class and they both love it because a few other grannies go, too.' Her eyes widened in horror. 'If one of them brought in some home-made snacks and sweetened them with honey instead of sugar, thinking it was healthier…'

'Your mum dotes on Noah,' Rob said. 'You know she'd never willingly let anything happen to him.'

'I'll call her now,' Lucy said. 'Do I need to go

into the corridor to use my phone? You know, so it doesn't interfere with any of the equipment?'

'You're fine in here,' Mo said. 'We'll give you both some space.'

Ten minutes later, Lucy came out of the relatives' room with Rob holding her hand and tears running down her cheeks. 'Mum says she went to her friend's for lunch after the class, and Noah ate half a cookie there. It never occurred to her to ask what was in it—Mum didn't eat one because she's on a diet—but it's the only thing she can think of that might've had honey in it. She rang her friend to ask her, and Mum just called me back to say yes, there was honey instead of sugar in the cookies.' She dragged in a breath. 'What's in honey that's made Noah ill like this?'

'Not *all* honey,' Mandy said, 'but some raw honey has been shown to contain botulin spores.'

'Botulin?' Rob looked horrified. 'But that kills people, doesn't it? Are you telling us that Noah's going to die?'

'No. He should make a full recovery, over the next couple of months,' Daniel said. 'A century ago, you're right, the outcome wouldn't have been so good; but thankfully medicine has advanced in this area. We can get some special infant antitoxin for him. We're going to talk to the pharmacy now, because we think it'll have to be shipped here from abroad.'

Lucy's eyes widened. 'Why isn't there any of this antitoxin stuff in a London hospital?'

'It's not a stock item because infant botulism is really rare in this country. It's less rare in America, so we'll contact the public health team in California that produces the antitoxin,' Mandy explained. 'We're going to test Noah's stools for the bacteria, but the lab results might take a few days. We won't wait for the results before we start treating him. The clinical diagnosis makes a lot of sense where his symptoms are concerned. Basically, the toxin stops the nerve endings telling the muscles to contract, so the first symptoms of the illness will be the baby finding it hard to suck or swallow, and being a bit constipated—which is what you reported.'

'Plus it doesn't cause a fever,' Mo said.

'This thing with the nerve endings—is that why Noah's floppy?' Lucy asked.

'Yes, and it's also why he might have trouble breathing,' Daniel said. 'We'll keep him in the coma for now, to keep him comfortable and support his breathing. It'll take him a little while to recover, because the nerve endings need to re-grow before they can send the right signals to his muscles; we'll need to give him support for breathing and feeding until he can do it himself, but over the next few weeks he'll get better.'

'And it won't affect him…the way he develops?' Rob asked.

'The toxin doesn't go into his brain or anything like that. He'll develop completely normally,' Mandy said. 'The only thing that will need to be delayed a bit are his immunisations, until six months after we've treated him, because the antitoxin would interfere with the live virus vaccinations—that's the MMR and varicella. We'll make sure your GP and health visitor know.'

'So he's going to be all right?' Lucy asked.

'He's going to be all right,' Mo confirmed.

'Thank God,' Lucy whispered. 'But right now I don't think I want Mum to look after him ever again.'

'It wasn't done deliberately, and your mum wasn't to know,' Daniel said gently. 'Remember, you're *her* baby, and my guess is she'll be in bits at the idea of being responsible for something that hurt your baby and therefore hurt you. Don't be too hard on her.'

'But if Dr Cooke here hadn't realised what it was, Noah might've become too ill to be treated,' Rob said. 'He might have…' He shook his head, clearly unable or unwilling to voice his deepest fears.

'I'm going to be a grannie in a few weeks' time,' Mandy said, 'and Dr Monroe's absolutely right in what he said. If I inadvertently do anything that hurts my daughter's baby, I'll never forgive myself for that—or for the pain and worry I caused my daughter. Your mum will be hugely upset about this, Lucy.'

'I don't have children,' Daniel added, 'but I have nieces and nephews, and I feel the same way about them.'

Something in his expression, quickly hidden, made Mandy wonder what he wasn't saying. Had it been his choice not to have children? Not that it was any of her business.

'You'll see Noah recover a little bit more every day,' Mo said. 'He'll need to be in hospital for a few weeks yet, but you can have as much involvement as you like in his care. The nurses will help you set up a routine. You'll be able to give him baths, feed him and cuddle him. Though for the next three months or so you'll need to be super-strict about handwashing after you've changed his nappy, because the toxins will come out in his faeces. If you've got an open cut on your hands, I'd wear gloves when you change him, to make sure the bacteria doesn't spread to you.'

'So we could catch it from Noah?' Rob asked.

'With an open wound, yes. But it won't affect you in the same way,' Mo said.

* * *

Once the Carmichaels were reassured that Noah would still be poorly for a little while but was going to make a good recovery, Daniel took Mandy to meet the pharmacy team.

'Baby botulism antitoxin? We'll definitely have to talk to California for that,' Navreen, the head of Pharmacy, said. 'Actually, this'll be good training for my team, because we haven't got well-established processes for getting something like this from abroad. We'll need to coordinate authorisation and Customs.'

'But you can definitely do it?' Mandy asked.

'We've done it a couple of times in the past. The systems have probably changed since the last time we did it; but don't worry, we'll get it sorted.' Navreen glanced at Daniel. 'Is this case going on your show?'

'Maybe,' Daniel said. 'I need to talk to the baby's mum and dad about it, but I think they could do with a bit of time to come to terms with what's happening before I ask their permission.'

Navreen nodded. 'If they say yes, we're happy for you to film here, too.'

'Great. Thank you.' He smiled at her. 'It'd be good to showcase other bits of the hospital, so the audience realises how wide our team is.' He gave her a hammy wink. 'Not just Dr Charming showing off and hogging the screen.'

Navreen laughed. 'Dan, we all know you're not like that.' She checked something on her computer. 'I was about to say the bad news is, we're eight hours ahead of California and we'll have to wait to get hold of them; but the good news is that their helpline is twenty-four-seven and we can call them now.' She glanced back at her screen. 'Though it looks as if you'll have to talk to their doctors about your clinical findings before they'll agree to let us have the antitoxin.'

'We can do that. Let's make the call,' Daniel said.

CHAPTER TWO

'WELL, THAT WAS a baptism of fire,' Daniel said, two hours later, finding them a quiet table in the hospital canteen and sliding the tray of their sandwiches and coffee onto it.

'At least now there's a procedure in place, if we ever get another patient with those symptoms,' Mandy said, 'even if it ends up needing to be tweaked in the future. The lab's extracting the toxins and culturing the faeces so we can isolate the bacteria, the public health authority is sending us the antitoxin, and we've got all the legal permissions in place to get it through Customs quickly.'

'And we can start treating baby Noah later today.' He took a sip of his coffee and closed his eyes briefly. 'Ahh. Just what I needed.' He opened his eyes again and looked at her. 'You said earlier that you're going to be a grandmother?'

'I don't really feel old enough,' she said. 'But,

when I look at it logically, Gemma's almost the same age I was when I had her.'

'Are you and your partner looking forward to the baby?' Oh, way to go, Daniel, he thought. Why not make it obvious that you're fishing? He blew out a breath. 'Sorry. That was intrusive and it's none of my business.'

'It's fine. Actually, there's just me,' she said.

Did that mean she was a widow? Divorced? Was Gemma's father not involved in her life at all? Not that he could ask. He'd already been pushy enough. And why was he so intrigued by her, in any case? He pushed the thought aside.

'And, yes, I'm looking forward to the baby arriving. Ten weeks, if he or she is on time.' Mandy raised an eyebrow. 'But you and I both know from experience that babies arrive when they're ready, and not when a calendar says they're supposed to.'

'Don't they just?' He couldn't help smiling at her. 'I remember my sister being furious when she went overdue with her first, and she got crosser by the day. In the end, she had to be in-duced. And even at the age of twenty-five my nephew's still very laid-back.'

'Have you got many nieces and nephews?' she asked.

'Four—my brother and sister both had one of each,' he said.

'You weren't tempted?' And then her face turned bright pink. 'Sorry. That was nosey. I apologise.'

He'd wanted children, all right. But he hadn't wanted to risk them turning out like him.

Like his father.

Not that he was going to tell Mandy any of that. He hadn't told anyone about those feelings, not even his mum and his siblings. 'You and I have only just met. How are we going to know anything about each other, unless we ask?' And if she asked him questions, he could ask her, too…

'That's true,' she said. 'Although I could say I know you from your TV show.'

'Tricky,' he said. 'If I say I'm just like I am on TV, that sounds a bit vain—and I can assure you, I'm not vain. The production team are forever waving a comb at me.' Though his sister teased him that having messy hair just attracted women who wanted to mother him. 'On the other hand, if I say I'm nothing like I am on TV, that makes me someone who can put on a false persona at will—which also isn't true.'

'The truth is that, like most people, you're somewhere in between,' she said. 'I admit, I assumed you were charming, like you are on the TV—and my mum's very fond of saying that charming is as charming does.'

Interestingly, Mandy's face went a little bit tight as she quoted her mum. So did she agree? Had she been hurt by someone charming—the father of her daughter, perhaps? 'We work in an area,' Daniel said, 'where the parents of our patients can get very, very anxious, very, very quickly. We need to be charming so we can put them at their ease and stop the panic spiralling enough for them to be able to breathe, think and listen to us. Then they can make an informed decision about their child's treatment, and let us get on with doing our job and making their child better.' He spread his hands. 'What's the use of a doctor who can't make eye contact, mumbles and sits with his back to the patient or their parents, tapping notes into a computer?'

'Much better to listen to the patients and their parents and look at them, so you can assess what kind of approach works best for them,' she said. 'That's not being charming. It's using your skills to do the best by your patient and showing them they can trust you.'

'I think they're one and the same,' he said. 'Is your definition of charming something that's surface and has no substance?'

'Yes,' she said.

He grinned. 'That's my definition of a politician.'

'You'll get no arguments from me, there,' she said.

Had her ex been a politician? he wondered. 'Well, I'm not a politician. In fact, you might have to kick me under my desk before a meeting with the suits and remind me that I have to play nice.'

'When really you're dying to ask why they need an antique desk instead of a perfectly serviceable flatpack desk, and point out that the price difference could go towards equipment to help our patients,' she said. 'If I kick you for that, you'll have to kick me as well.'

'A woman after my own heart—as well as being a bringer of brownies. We're going to get on fine as job-shares,' he said.

'Even if I turn up wearing an eye patch with sequins tomorrow?'

'Like a pirate?' He couldn't help laughing. '"Dr Cooke" rhymes with "Captain Hook", you know.'

She groaned. 'I walked straight into that one, didn't I?'

'You're seriously going to have a sequinned eye patch tomorrow?'

'Gemma's planning to do it as the craft session at school today—at least, that's what she threatened, this morning. She teaches Reception class,' Mandy explained with a smile.

Clearly they had a close relationship, and he pushed down the little twinge of envy. He'd made his decision, years ago, and he knew it had been the right one. Even if he did feel sometimes that he'd missed out.

'So what else did you want to ask me?' she asked.

'We could always start with the one everyone uses at conferences—what made you pick your specialty?'

'Paediatrics was my favourite rotation. I like how quickly children respond to treatment and start getting better,' she said promptly. 'You?'

'Same,' he said. 'I nearly stayed with obstetrics, because that moment when a new life comes into the world is so special. But generally the jokes from our patients are more on my level.' He raised his eyebrows at her. 'Why did the bicycle lean against the wall?'

'Do your worst, Dr Monroe,' she said, putting her hands on her hips and fixing him with an amused stare.

'Because it was two-tyred.' He mimed playing drums and crashing a cymbal.

She groaned and then laughed, and Daniel realised just how pretty she was. It felt as if she'd just lit up the room, and it caused another of those weird swoopy feelings in his stomach.

'Can I pass that one on to Gemma for her class?' she asked.

'Be my guest. And I'm all ears if you have a secret stash of bad jokes,' he added.

'The cheesier, the "grater"?' she asked.

He grinned. That terrible pun made him like her even more. 'It'd Brie rude not to share,' he said back.

Her eyes crinkled at the corners. 'I suppose it's Feta to let you have the last word.'

'That'd be really Gouda,' he said, unable to help himself.

This was work. They were meant to be talking about serious things. But everything about Amanda Cooke made him want to smile and have fun.

'I think we've done enough cheese jokes,' she said, though he rather thought she sounded rueful instead of bossy. 'What made you become a TV doctor?'

'I fell into it pretty much by accident,' he admitted. 'A friend volunteered me to help another friend with the pitch she was writing for the series—telling her about the kind of cases we treat here. She got a slot for the pitch and asked me to go to the studio with her to answer questions on the medical side. At the end of the pitch, the producer said I had a good voice for TV. The next thing I knew, I was talking to the CEO of the London Victoria about whether we'd be prepared to film the show here, and if I could fit filming round my job.'

'Clearly the answer was yes, as it's been running for five years now,' she said.

'I've been lucky,' he said. 'I never expected to enjoy it so much. And the best bit for me is getting letters from viewers—when someone's been really struggling to get a diagnosis for their child, sees a similar case on the show, and then puts it all together and finally manages to get the help they need. Hearing that the show's been able to make a real difference to a child's health is just brilliant.'

'Is that why you showcase case studies with common conditions as well as the rarer ones?' she asked.

'Definitely. We always have a bronchiolitis case in every series. I remember my first winter as a junior doctor in Paediatrics; I walked in one morning to see a whole bay of poorly babies all on oxygen therapy, with a laminated note on their door warning "RSV+"—it really shocked me, especially when the nurses told me I needed to use extra protective clothing before I went in to check them on my ward round, so I didn't spread the virus to the rest of the ward. That hadn't even occurred to me. And seeing them all struggling...' He grimaced. 'It's always harder for the tinier ones.'

'Because their airways are so small, they get gummed up more quickly and they're also more likely to develop pneumonia,' Mandy agreed. 'And it's really scary for the parents when their baby's too tired to feed and they need feeding through a nasogastric tube.'

'I've had letters from people who were sure their baby had more than just a bad cold, but at the same time they didn't want to bother the doctor with something trivial. Thanks to the show, they could see what intercostal recession actually looked like, and it prompted them to take the baby to their family doctors and get the right help,' he said. 'And it's also comforting to parents who are worried sick about their baby being on oxygen therapy and fed through a nasogastric tube; the show reassures them that it's standard treatment, loads of babies get the virus every year, and they really will get better.'

'I'm all for reassurance,' she said.

He'd already gathered that. It was another one of the things he really liked about his new colleague. He'd never felt so in tune with anyone in his life.

Daniel opened his mouth to ask her if maybe she'd like to have dinner with him, and thankfully stopped himself just in time. Was he insane? They'd only just met. Asking her to dinner would send completely the wrong message. He didn't believe in relationships and it really wouldn't be a good idea to have a fling with his new job-share. The last thing they needed was things to become awkward between them, which of course they would when the fling was over.

He'd simply have to keep his usual pleasant, professional distance from her and damp down that flare of attraction he felt, because it couldn't go anywhere.

Instead, he switched the conversation back to a safe topic: work, and her training plans. 'So how did you end up teaching?'

'Pure accident. I stepped in for a colleague who was off sick and hated the training aspect of the job in any case because he didn't have much patience with students. I discovered I loved it—I enjoyed their energy and enthusiasm, and they all liked the way I worked with them. They asked me quietly if there was any chance I could keep teaching them when my colleague came back. I had a chat with my colleague and he agreed. It worked for all of us.'

Daniel wasn't surprised her students had responded to her in that way. Just from seeing the way she'd interacted with the team in the intensive care unit and the pharmacy, he'd realised she was supportive and enabling. 'That's so good when that happens,' Daniel said. 'I love the energy and enthusiasm of students, too. And I never mind questions, either; we've all been in a place where we don't have a clue. And I'd much rather someone asked me the same question ten times than panicked, guessed and got it wrong.' He glanced at his watch. 'We need to get back. And hopefully by now the estates team have put another desk and computer in our office, which was supposed to happen last week, and your staff card's turned up.'

Mandy left the hospital after her shift with a smile on her face. She liked her new colleagues and the way the team worked together.

The only thing that worried her was her reaction to Daniel Monroe. She'd found herself instantly connecting with him—they shared similar values and a similar sense of humour. She'd liked the way he'd reassured the Carmichaels, supported Mo and clearly had a good working relationship with the pharmacy team. He was a dream colleague.

But.

She'd also found herself reacting to him as a woman. Responding to his warmth and charm. Even though she'd learned the hard way from her marriage that charm was the flip side of unreliability and selfishness, her libido had prac-

tically sat up and begged at the first smile from
Dr TWC.

And that made him dangerous.

Her smile faded.

Even if he was interested—and by no means
was she going to assume that the attraction she
felt towards him was mutual—she didn't have
room in her life for a relationship. When Gemma
was small, Mandy had been too busy to date,
unable to find the time between the demands of
parenting and the crazy hours of a junior doctor. By the time Gemma was a teenager, Mandy
had learned how to deflect the question before it
was even asked, and made it clear to any seem-
ingly interested male that the only relationship
she was interested in was friendship. But now...?

Now, she'd just need to make sure those defences stayed in place whenever she was around
Daniel.

On the way to Gemma's, she texted her mum,
her sister and her best friend to confirm that her
first day had been fabulous and she'd got on well
with all her new colleagues.

Her sister texted back.

What about the sexy TV doctor?

Mandy replied firmly.

Nice guy and will be a good colleague.

She answered her mum's and best friend's questions in the same vein.

And then it was time to face Gemma.

'Mum, your eye looks so *sore*.' Gemma hugged her.

'I'm fine,' Mandy said lightly. 'Something smells delicious, Dev.'

Her son-in-law smiled. 'Perfect timing. Dinner's ready in five minutes.'

'Something for you, Mum.' Gemma gave her a small parcel wrapped in tissue paper.

Mandy groaned, pretty sure she knew what was in it: and, just as she suspected, when she opened it she found a pink eye patch covered with silver sequins and bordered with lace.

'My class wants a picture of you in your white coat, wearing it,' Gemma said.

'I don't wear a white coat,' Mandy said. 'But all right, I'll take it to work tomorrow and take a selfie with this and my stethoscope.'

'Atta-Mum,' Gemma said. 'Seriously, tell me all about your day.'

'Wait for me!' Dev called from the kitchen. 'I'm dishing up now.'

Over dinner, Mandy told them about her day.

'Does this mean you might end up on TV, too?' Dev asked.

'Possibly,' Mandy said.

'That's cool,' Devi said.

'And what's Dr Monroe like in the flesh?' Gemma asked.

'Calm, capable and kind,' Mandy said.

Gemma raised an eyebrow. 'You're blushing.'

'Don't be ridiculous,' Mandy said, even though she could feel the colour seeping into her face.

'So he's as gorgeous in real life as he is on the screen?'

'Like a lot of actors are,' Mandy said. 'Except Dan's a proper doctor.'

Gemma eyed her thoughtfully. 'You know, if he's a nice guy and he's single, you think he's attractive and he likes you too—and of course he'll like you, because you're the loveliest person I know—there's no reason why you can't date him.'

'I can tell you one, straight off: he's my colleague,' Mandy said.

'Plenty of people meet at work,' Dev said. 'It's not a barrier.'

'I don't have time,' Mandy said.

'Maybe you need to make time, Mum,' Gemma said gently.

'I'm happy with the family and friends I already have. I don't need a relationship,' Mandy protested.

Yet the idea lodged in her head, and despite trying to ignore it she found herself thinking about Daniel all the way home.

Even if he was as attracted to her as she was to him, dating him wouldn't be sensible.

But she'd spent a lifetime being sensible. And, even though she'd refused to admit it to Gemma, she did have moments where she felt lonely. Moments when she wished she had someone to share her life with. Even if it was only for a little while.

She'd see how things went, this week. And then maybe…

By the end of the week, Mandy felt as if she'd been working at the London Victoria for ever. Baby Noah was still in Intensive Care and still needed support for his breathing, but the antitoxin had arrived safely from America and his treatment had started. Khaj had introduced her to Hayley, the teenager with cystic fibrosis who loved sewing, and Mandy had brought in a complicated embroidery pattern for Hayley and taught her the stiches during her lunchbreak. She was really enjoying working with her students—and with Daniel. He was more than just the charming doctor he seemed to be on the television; he really did care about their patients. So maybe he was the exception: a charming man who was actually reliable.

'Are you doing anything nice tonight?' he asked on Friday afternoon, when they were both finalising the last bits of paperwork towards the end of their shift.

'Yes—it's my ballet class on Fridays,' she said with a smile. 'It's the highlight of my week.'

He tipped his head to one side. 'Thinking about it, you do move like a dancer. Graceful,' he said. 'I can just see you in a—not a tutu, but one of those floaty long skirts.'

Mandy felt tell-tale heat flood into her cheeks. 'Thank you. The class is for older adult beginners; I've been doing it for four years, now. Having to remember the choreography's really good for my synapses.'

'It's good for flexibility and balance, too,' Daniel said. 'Plus mental health—if you're concentrating on the movement, you don't have headspace to think about anything else and you can switch off.'

'I always feel lighter of spirit, afterwards,' she admitted. 'The way you just talked about it, it sounds as if you do ballet classes, too?'

'No. I count reps in the gym, which does the same sort of thing for my mental health,' he said. 'Obviously the music I use in the gym's a bit faster, but I listen to ballet music when I want to chill out. And I've been known to accompany someone to the ballet.'

Of course he had. Probably a prima ballerina,

she thought. Someone as gorgeous as Daniel would always have a beautiful companion.

It must've been written in her expression, because he said, 'My youngest niece, for her sixth birthday,' he said. 'I took Daisy and my sister to see a matinee of *The Nutcracker*. She was spellbound—I wasn't sure what I enjoyed watching most, the show or the sheer joy on her face.'

Yet again he'd wrongfooted her. This wasn't about him being a celebrity dating another celebrity; it was about family. 'That's a lovely thing to do.'

'I take my duties as an uncle very seriously. I want to be part of their lives and spend proper time with them, doing things they love,' he said. 'Whether it's an afternoon at the park, pushing them on a swing, reading a gazillion stories, making cupcakes with glitter sprinkles or a big birthday treat like going to the ballet. Or sitting drinking a glass of wine with them, now they're older.'

The fact he'd enjoyed spending time with the children in his family really struck a chord with her: it was just as she'd done with Gemma. 'Making memories is important,' she said. 'How old are they now?'

'Daisy's twenty-two; she started off studying medicine, but she really hated it and she switched to train in music therapy, which suits her a lot better. Her brother James is twenty-five; he's an archaeologist and still likes dragging me mudlarking on a Sunday morning, if the tide's right,' he said, smiling fondly. 'Milo, my brother's son, is also twenty-five; he's in software development and loves gadgets, and his elder sister Hannah is twenty-eight and has just qualified as a GP.'

He sounded as proud of them as if they were his own children; to her secret delight, he took out his phone and scrolled through some snaps before handing it to her. 'That's them after Daisy's graduation.'

The photograph was of four young adults, all dressed up and with their arms around each other, with a background of a flower wall. 'That's lovely.'

'We had dinner with them; then they all went off clubbing with Daisy's mates while we went back to Ally's—Daisy's mum's—for champagne and cheese.'

'That sounds like what we did for Gemma's graduation. A family meal out to celebrate, then sending her off for cocktails and clubbing with her friends.' She smiled. 'Are you doing anything special, this weekend?'

'Supper and a grilling at my parents' place, tomorrow night, with the whole family,' he said cheerfully. 'They'll want to know all about my new job-share, and if she might be suitable for sharing more than my job.'

Mandy's eyes widened. 'Seriously?'

'I'm very tempted to tease them and tell them you're a goddess and I've begged you on my bended knees to date me, but you're utterly heartless and won't take pity on me.' He grinned. 'But I'll resist the temptation, because I know that'd blow up in my face. My sister and my sister-in-law would make an excuse to drop in and grill you as to exactly what you think's wrong with me and why you haven't accepted a date with me. So I'll just tell them the truth. It feels as if you've always been part of the team, you brought in home-made cake on your first day and I'm rather hoping that's going to be a Monday morning thing in the future, and you're absolutely not in the market for hanging around with a reprobate like me.'

She wasn't quite sure how to react to that. Being single, did he get the same worried inquisition that she did from her own family about when she was going to settle down, and he was making light of it? Was he teasing about wanting to maybe date her? Or had he secretly been thinking the same thing that she had—that her new colleague was very easy on the eye, made the day feel brighter, and over this last week she'd discovered that she really looked forward to coming into work and seeing him?

'Don't forget to tell them that I have a better stock of terrible jokes than you do,' she said, deciding to take it all as teasing.

'That's rampant cheating, because your daughter teaches Reception class and that gives you an unfair advantage,' he retorted. 'But I suppose you have a point. What about you—are you seeing your family at the weekend?'

'My best friend goes to ballet class with me, and I'm seeing my mum and my sister tomorrow for dinner,' she said. 'They'll all want to know if you're the same in real life as you are on TV. I'll tell them that you're probably better, because you always listen to the nurses and you've got time for the patients and their parents.'

'That's nice,' he said. 'Better than I am on TV. I like that.' His eyes glittered. 'Seems that we have quite a mutual admiration society going on here.'

They did. But it wasn't going anywhere further than friendship.

'Well, have a lovely weekend, Ms Cooke,' he said.

'You, too, Mr Monroe.' She sketched him a bow.

CHAPTER THREE

'DAN, ARE YOU ever going to settle down?' his sister asked, pushing a dish of apple crumble in his direction and indicating to him to add his own custard.

'I'm already settled, Ally,' he said, giving her his sweetest smile. 'If I went any higher at the hospital, I'd be stuck in a suit's job doing nothing but meetings and never seeing a patient, which isn't why I became a doctor. I love my job just as it is. Plus I've lived in the same house for ten years. I don't think I can get more settled than that.'

She narrowed her eyes at him. 'You know what I mean. It's half a lifetime since you split up with Roxy.'

'I'm too busy to date, between the hospital and the TV show and spending time with my favourite people—which, strangely enough, is you lot, despite all the nagging,' he said lightly.

'What about your new colleague? Is she nice?' Sasha, his sister-in-law, put in.

'You mean, is she available?' He rolled his eyes. 'I knew you'd all start. I told Mandy exactly what you'd say—and I'll tell you what I told her. It feels as if she's always been part of the team, she brought in home-made chocolate cake on her first day to introduce herself to everyone, and even if I was in the market for a relationship, she's not.'

'She's married, then.' His mother looked disappointed.

Not any more, but they didn't need to know that. He looked at his brother and brother-in-law. 'Um, a little male solidarity, here, please, guys? Call them off?'

'You're on your own, mate,' Jake, his brother-in-law, said.

'It's more than my life's worth,' Colin, his brother, added.

'Scandalous,' Daniel said, sighing, and poured custard over his apple crumble. 'Now, let's talk about something more interesting than my love life. Which, as I've been telling you for a very long time, isn't going to change any time soon.'

Though he had to acknowledge later that night that the idea had lodged in his head.

Amanda Cooke.

He liked her. A lot. She had a warmth people couldn't help responding to, a sense of humour that was similar to his own, and he'd caught her taking a selfie in her office for her daughter's class, wearing her stethoscope and the pink sequin and lace eye patch they'd made for her. She was a woman who noticed the little things, and she'd learned the names of everyone on the ward within two days, regardless of their role on the team.

And there was no denying that she was attractive. He wished he hadn't thought about her wearing a floaty chiffon ballet skirt, because he couldn't get that picture out of his head: a graceful pirouette towards him with her skirt swishing round, and then he'd catch her round the waist and...

Oh, for pity's sake. She'd made it clear she wasn't interested in him other than as a colleague. He had no intention of ruining their professional relationship; he'd learned a very hard lesson when his marriage had disintegrated. So he'd just have to stuff these little flutters of awareness back into their box and ignore them.

On Monday, Mandy left home-made cookies on Daniel's desk, wrapped in greaseproof paper and with a note.

Happy Monday, dear Job-share ☺

But her bright mood disappeared fast when she did the ward round with her students and came to three-week-old baby Aarya, who'd been admitted with scarlet fever caused by Group A Streptococcus.

'Group A Strep's quite common,' she said. 'Usually it causes a sore throat and a fever, but not a runny nose or a cough. You might see white spots on the back of the baby's throat and they'll be poorly for a few days. Can anyone tell me what it sometimes leads to?'

'Scarlet fever?' one of the students suggested.

'Yes,' Mandy said. 'What can you tell me about scarlet fever?'

'It makes a child's tongue and lips go red, and they get a red pinprick rash all over their bodies,' another said.

'Starting where?' Mandy asked.

'The trunk, and then it spreads to the arms and legs,' another said.

'Can you see a rash on baby Aarya?' Mandy asked.

'No,' one of the others said.

'It's harder to see the rash on brown skin. So how else can you check?' Mandy asked.

'The skin feels like sandpaper?' one of the students asked.

She nodded. 'What would you recommend for treatment?'

'Antibiotics for the bacterial infection, and liquid paracetamol for the fever,' one of the students said.

'Good. Anything else you'd suggest?'

'Keep the baby home for the first twenty-four hours, to stop it spreading?' another student said.

'Yes. Scarlet fever's a notifiable disease,' she said, 'so you also need to let the local health protection team know; and give the mum penicillin as well, as a precaution. And remember to check for penicillin allergy before you prescribe the antibiotics.'

She got them to talk through how scarlet fever spread, the incubation period and how long an affected child would be infectious, the possible complications, and which groups were most at risk. Most of them knew that most cases occurred in the under-tens, and the most common age for children to get it was four.

What worried her was that Aarya was in a really high-risk group because of her age.

'Most babies with GAS throat infection recovery quickly with antibiotics,' she said, 'but rare cases turn into iGAS—invasive Group A Strep. The virus decreases the baby's ability to fight off the infection, which spreads through the bloodstream and releases toxins into the body, and that can lead to organ failure and, in the worst-case scenario, the baby doesn't make it. Hopefully that's not going to be the case here.' But the baby's notes told her that the GP had already given antibiotics, two days before, and Aarya's temperature was still sky-high.

She led the students through the rest of the ward round, assessing their knowledge, but between ward rounds and clinic she popped back to see the baby.

A woman who looked to be in her early thirties was sitting next to the baby's tiny cot, holding her hand.

'You must be Aarya's mum,' Mandy said.

'Yes. Neelam Chakrabarti,' the younger woman confirmed.

'Hello, Neelam. I'm Mandy Cooke, one of the ward doctors,' Mandy said. 'I saw Aarya when I did ward rounds earlier—thank you, by the way, for agreeing to let my students see her, too. How are you doing?'

'Not great,' Neelam admitted. 'Nish, her dad, was called into work, or he'd be here as well.'

'It's tough when your little one's in hospital,' Mandy said. 'Is there anyone else I can call for you who can give you some support?'

'No.' A tear trickled down her face, and she wiped it away. 'I just wish I could take this from Aarya.'

Mandy, who'd felt the same over the years when her own daughter had been ill, reached over to squeeze her hand. 'She's in the right place. How long has she had the rash?'

'Three days. I didn't think she was well last week, because she was fussy and refusing to feed and had a runny nose. I thought it was a cold. Then her temperature went up, and I couldn't get it down. The GP said it might be a streptococcus infection, because it was doing the rounds, and he gave her antibiotics. When the rash started, the doctors here said it was scarlet fever.'

'Strep A can cause scarlet fever,' Mandy said. 'Did the doctor give you antibiotics as well?'

'When I went back to see him, after the rash started and I still couldn't get her temperature down, he said I should take the antibiotics too and see how Aarya's doing in a couple of days.' She bit her lip. 'I know the hospital's busy and you don't need the extra patients fussing, but...'

'You did exactly the right thing, bringing her in,' Mandy reassured her. 'Babies can become so ill, so quickly. I never mind seeing a baby who's got something really minor and I can re-assure the parents it's nothing to worry about. I know it's scary, being in hospital, but it means we can keep an eye on her and treat her quickly if anything changes.'

'I know where it started. My friend's little boy had a bit of a cold,' Neelam said, brushing away another tear. 'She wanted to come and see the baby. It was only for a few minutes, on the way home from the childminder. She feels terrible that he might have given her this.'

'If you give me her details,' Mandy said, 'I'll give her a quick call and ask her to get him checked over by her GP in case he develops scarlet fever, too, and let her childminder know to tell her other clients, just to be on the safe side.'

'All right,' Neelam said. 'Her number's in my phone.'

'Whenever you've got a moment,' Mandy said. 'Is there anything you want to ask me?'

'How long will it take until her temperature comes down?'

'A fever's a sign that her body's fighting an infection,' Mandy said. 'Usually a fever will break on the fourth or fifth day. The main thing is to keep her comfortable and well hydrated. Right now she's too tired to feed and struggling a bit with breathing, which is why she's on a nasogastric tube and oxygen therapy.'

'I'm expressing milk for her,' Neelam said.

'Which is great, plus you're here with her— she can hear your voice and feel you holding her hand. That'll help to comfort and calm her,' Mandy said. 'But you also need to look after yourself, Neelam. If you're tired and need a break, please take some time. We'll keep a close eye on her here.'

'I just want to be with her,' Neelam said.

'I understand that,' Mandy said gently. 'My daughter's due to have her first baby in a couple of months and it's very hard not to call her all the time, just to check on her.'

'So you never stop worrying, as a mum?'

Mandy gave a wry smile. 'No. Your worries just change. But the love makes up for it.' She checked the baby's charts. 'Someone in the team will be popping in very regularly to see how she's doing, but please come and find one of us if you're worried about anything at all. That's what we're here for.'

'I will,' Neelam promised.

Mandy dropped in to the office she shared with Daniel and was relieved to see him there at his desk.

'Good morning, Mandy, and thank you for the cookies,' he said. 'I was teasing—I really don't expect you to bake every Sunday and bring me goodies every Monday morning—but thank you. They were appreciated.'

'Pleasure,' she said. 'I know you're busy, but there's a case I really think we need to keep an eye on.' She gave him a quick rundown on baby Aarya. 'Especially as she's so young, I'm worried about that GAS infection.'

'Good call,' he said. 'I'll keep a check. How are the students?'

'I think they enjoyed ward rounds. There's one of them I think will make an exceptional doctor. Anyway, I've got them paired off for clinic next—including one with me, so I'll get going.'

'I'll keep you up to date with the baby,' he said.

'Thank you. I appreciate it,' she said.

'And remember,' he said quietly, 'it's rare.'

He'd clearly picked up on her secret worry: that something might happen to Gemma and Dev's baby. 'I know,' she said, hoping that the wobble didn't show in her voice.

Even though she was busy with clinic, she was half expecting to be called out during it. It overran slightly, so at lunchtime she had just enough time to gulp down a sandwich and a coffee and to see Aarya, who appeared to be holding her own.

But then, late afternoon, she was called to a crash team. Baby Aarya's blood pressure had dropped rapidly, due to the infection, her oxygen saturations had also dropped, and she'd gone into arrest.

Daniel was already there, managing the neonate's airway. Neelam and a man Mandy guessed was her husband Nish were also present; another of the nurses was clearly explaining what was going on and making sure that they didn't distract the resuscitation team.

'I've just given Aarya the adrenaline,' Daniel said.

Mandy's training kicked in, ignoring the fact that this was a three-week-old baby in trouble. The important thing now was to get that heart beating again. 'I'll bag,' she said. Daniel held the mask in place while she gave the baby twenty-five breaths per minute. In the meantime, Khaj had put the ECG leads in place.

'Asystole,' Khaj said, glancing at the monitor.

Daniel and Mandy exchanged a glance. The baby's heart still wasn't beating, and they could only shock the heart if it was a case of pulseless ventricular tachycardia or ventricular fibrillation. Any other rhythm wasn't shockable.

'Khaj, hold the mask in place for me, please,' Daniel said. 'Mandy, keep bagging. I'll start the compressions.'

He pushed down on the baby's chest, counting out loud.

'Two minutes—swap,' Mandy said, and continued the fast compressions, counting them while Daniel took over bagging.

Still no response.

'Come on, Aarya. You can do it,' he whispered fiercely.

At the end of the two-minute cycle, Mandy administered adrenaline again.

'Still asystole,' Khaj said.

'Swap,' Mandy said, and did the bagging while Daniel did the compressions.

Two more cycles, another bolus of adrenaline, and still nothing.

'Keep going,' Daniel said.

Two more cycles of CPR, more adrenaline, and still nothing.

They worked for twenty more minutes.

Finally, Daniel shook his head. 'I'm sorry, everyone. She's not responding. I'm going to call it, now. I'm so sorry.'

Neelam wailed in grief and clutched at her husband.

Mandy knew that having the parents there while a child was being resuscitated was painful, but at the same time it would be comforting later because they could see for themselves that the team had done everything they could.

Gently, she stroked the baby's face. 'I'm so sorry, little one,' she whispered. She walked over to the Chakrabartis and hugged them both. 'I'm so very, very sorry.'

'She can't be gone. She *can't* be!' Nish said, his voice cracking with tension.

'I'm sorry.' Mandy knew how inadequate the words were.

'It happened so fast—one second she was fine, and the next there were alarms going off and...' Neelam shook her head. 'I can't...' Her words faded and she just looked numb.

'Group A Strep infections can be nasty,' Mandy said. 'Because she's so young, Aarya had fewer defences against it.'

'It caused her blood pressure to drop,' Daniel said, joining them, 'and some of her organs went into failure, including her heart. We tried our best, but we couldn't get her back.'

'Why didn't you do that thing everyone sees on the TV? Why didn't you shock her heart?' Nish asked.

'We can only shock a heart that's in a certain type of rhythm,' Daniel explained. 'Asystole is where the heart muscle doesn't contract, there's no electrical activity in the heart, and no blood flow to the rest of the body. Giving adrenaline, chest compressions and breathing for her, like we did, can sometimes restart the heart and get a different rhythm going, so then we'd be able to shock the heart, but it doesn't always work. I'm sorry. We tried our hardest.'

'It was only a cold,' Neelam whispered. 'She's not supposed to die from a *cold*.'

'I'm so sorry,' Mandy said yet again, knowing how inadequate it was but unable to find any other words to say.

Khaj came over to them. 'Would you like me to bring Aarya over to you so you can sit with her for a while?' she asked. 'We can clear the room so you have time with your daughter on your own.'

'Our little girl,' Nish said. 'We loved her so much. She was only three weeks old.' His eyes filled with tears. 'This doesn't seem possible. Why her? Why now?'

There weren't any answers to his questions. Just a wall of sadness and grief.

'Come and sit with Aarya,' Khaj said. 'It'll help you to be with her. We can contact the hospital chaplain to come in and say a prayer with you, if you'd like that.'

'I…' Neelam shook her head, looking dazed and as if she couldn't process anything.

'You don't have to decide anything now,' Mandy said gently. 'You've got all the time you need. If you want us to call someone for you, just tell us and we'll do it.'

'Anything you need, just tell us,' Daniel said.

'I think, right now, we just want to be on our own with our daughter,' Nish said.

The rest of Mandy's clinic felt like a blur. At the end of her shift, she went into her office. Daniel was there, looking grim.

'Are you OK?' he asked, glancing up at her.

'No,' she said. 'And you don't look OK, either.'

'I'm very far from OK,' he said. 'Losing any

patient is hard. But a three-week-old baby, and the way we lost her...' He blew out a breath. 'Khaj contacted the chaplain to come and see them, and I've given the Chakrabartis details of a bereavement counsellor and a support group. Though it doesn't feel like doing anything near enough.'

She knew exactly what he meant. She felt the same way. 'We tried our best. We all wanted a good outcome. But invasive Group A Strep can be a seriously nasty thing. Overwhelming. Intellectually, I know there was nothing more we could've done. But it still feels s—' She cut the word off, slumped into her chair and closed her eyes for a moment. 'I can't face going to my book group tonight. I'm not fit for anyone's company. I'm going to cancel.'

'I can't face people tonight, either,' Daniel said. 'Look, do you want to go for a walk with me? We don't have to talk—just put one foot in front of the other and keep each other company, on the grounds that it might help to decompress with someone else who's just been through what happened today.'

She thought about it. If she went home on her own, she'd brood. If Gemma rang her, she'd pick up on the fact Mandy wasn't her normal self. And Mandy absolutely couldn't tell her heavily pregnant daughter what had upset her so much. 'All right. That'd be good.'

'Give me twenty minutes to finish my paperwork?'

'Sure,' she said. 'Cup of tea?'

'You're an angel,' he said gratefully. 'Yes, please.'

While Mandy was waiting for the kettle to boil, she messaged her book club with an anodyne excuse; she managed to find some biscuits in the staff room, and came back with the spoils.

'Thank you,' Daniel said, though the strain around his eyes was obvious.

And although they both slogged through their paperwork, Mandy knew that neither of them was finding it easy. She was pretty sure that Daniel was thinking the same as she was: of the Chakrabatis, and how the light had gone out of their world. How their team had tried so very hard to save little Aarya, but they hadn't been able to start her heart again because the bacterial infection had been just too much for her tiny body to fight off.

Eventually, Daniel sighed. 'I think I'm going to come in early tomorrow to finish this lot. Right now, I can't concentrate.'

'Same here,' she admitted. 'Shall we just *go*?'

'Yes,' he said. 'After you went back to your clinic, I made sure the others weren't going to be on their own when they went home tonight. I'm going to do a proper debrief tomorrow, when we've all had a chance to get some rest and it doesn't feel quite as raw as it does now. Logically, I know we did everything we could. Just, in my heart, I keep wondering, what if we'd tried for another five minutes?' His face twisted.

'She wouldn't have survived. Her brain had already been too starved of oxygen. But I know what you mean. Me, too,' she said. 'Come on. We need those endorphins. Let's have that walk.'

CHAPTER FOUR

IT WASN'T QUITE dark when they left the hospital, but it was a grey and chilly autumn evening, and Mandy was glad of her coat.

'Shall we head for the river?' Daniel asked.

'Good idea,' she agreed.

Although they didn't speak as they trudged through the streets, it wasn't an awkward silence: more that neither of them could quite bear anything resembling a normal conversation just yet, and they took quiet comfort from each other's presence. A couple of times, their hands accidentally brushed; the third time it happened, Daniel took her hand.

It wasn't a clumsy attempt at a pass; she knew that he was simply offering her the comfort that she really needed, right then. He clearly needed that same comfort, so she walked hand in hand with him rather than pulling away. Funny how the warmth of his skin against hers made everything hurt just a little bit less. She hoped it was working for him, too.

When they reached the River Thames, they stood watching the traffic move over Chelsea Bridge for a while; the lights on the suspension bridge were reflected in the darkening water of the river.

'It's pretty in summer,' Daniel said. 'I usually walk to work this way.'

'You live in Chelsea?' Mandy asked.

'Round the corner from the Physic Garden. Which is always a lovely place to go,' he said. 'Where are you based?'

'I have a flat in King's Cross,' she said. 'In a gorgeous Georgian building.'

'Snap—well, mine's a townhouse. I had the chance of buying a modern flat overlooking the river,' he said, 'but I much prefer old buildings. They've got so much more character.'

Another area where they chimed, Mandy thought. She was starting to feel really in tune with Daniel—more than she had with anyone else she'd ever met. Which was unexpected, and also slightly unsettling.

'Shall we keep walking?' he asked.

She nodded, and they strolled alongside the river.

'Chelsea Hospital gardens are over there,' he said, indicating the other side of the road. 'That's my route home during summer, because it's open until sunset—well, obviously it's closed during the Chelsea Flower Show, too. But it's nice to have a green space so close.'

'I know what you mean,' she said. 'There are lots of pockets of little gardens near me, too, or I can walk down to the canal and the park at Camley Street. As you say, it's nice to walk through green spaces in summer.'

Still holding hands, they walked by the river down to the Albert Bridge and leaned against the embankment wall under one of the streetlamps, looking across the Thames.

'Did you know, apart from Tower Bridge, this is the only bridge in central London that's never been replaced?' he asked. 'And it's the only one with its original tollbooths—as well as a sign telling troops to break step when they walk over it. Apparently, if the men had marched in step, there's a chance the bridge would've collapsed.'

'It's that fragile?' she asked.

'Yes, but it gets patched up every so often,' he said. 'I like this bit of London. Henry VIII's old manor house gardens are just round the corner, with mulberry trees allegedly planted by Elizabeth I, and there are all the statues and monuments tucked along the embankment. Not to mention all the wisteria in the spring, and the gorgeous tree full of blossom outside St Luke's—where Dickens got married.'

Clearly he was distracting himself by dredging up facts and figures; though it was helping to distract her, too. 'There's so much of London I haven't explored,' she said. 'I really must make the effort.'

'In a job like ours, there isn't time to do much outside seeing your family,' he said. 'Especially in the early years.'

'Yes.' She bit her lip. 'When Gemma was born, I used to worry so much about her. Every sniffle took me back to being a second-year medical student, convinced that I'd developed the symptoms of whichever disease we'd covered that week—except this time I was convinced *she* was the one who'd developed those diseases.'

He gave her a wry smile. 'I remember being like that as a student, too. I think we were all hypochondriacs, those first couple of years.'

'Weren't we just? As a parent, I worried myself sick. As a grandparent, I think I'll be as bad,' she said. 'But what happened today…that's made it feel a hundred times worse. What if I go to see Gemma and the baby, and I don't even realise I've picked up a virus?' The idea almost made her hyperventilate with terror. 'What if I pass RSV to the baby, or Group A Strep, when she's still so tiny it'll overwhelm her system?'

'RSV's very possible, even if you use the extra PPE,' he said. 'But you already know we can do a lot for that particular virus, and anyway you won't go to see the baby if you've got what feels like a super-heavy cold because you're experienced enough to know what it is. And you're really not very likely to pick up Group A Str—oh, come *here*.' He wrapped his arms round her and held her close, resting his cheek against her hair. 'It's going to be OK, Mandy. Today was horrific, but how often does this happen?'

'It's rare,' she admitted. 'But it still feels horrible.'

'I know. But know also you did everything you could. We all did.'

It was a long, long time since a man had wrapped his arms round her, offering her comfort, Mandy thought. Not since her dad had died, five years ago. And if she didn't include her dad it had been even longer. Laurence, her ex, had never comforted her like this when she came home from a tough shift, tired and out of sorts; usually he'd been grumbling about having to miss a social event with his friends or colleagues because she was at work. Until he'd started going to them on his own…

She ought to pull away from Daniel. Now. For the sake of her own sanity. She wasn't going to let herself rely on a man, ever again.

Yet the bleakness in Daniel's expression when

he'd called the time of death on the baby made her think that he, too, needed the comfort of a cuddle. He'd made her feel better; she should do the same for him. So, instead of extracting herself with a feeble excuse, she wrapped her own arms around him. Held him close.

They stood there for a long, long moment, saying nothing, just holding each other.

Then she tipped her head back.

Whatever she'd been about to say was lost to the London evening, because his eyes were oh, so dark and all the words went out of her head. His mouth was very slightly parted. She could see the beginnings of a beard on his face; and, unable to stop herself, she reached up to glide her fingertips across his skin, feeling the catch of stubble.

Daniel sucked in a breath.

And then he twisted his head so his mouth brushed her palm. His lips were warm and soft, and she ached to feel them against hers.

Crazy, crazy, crazy.

This shouldn't be happening.

But now it had started, she couldn't stop it. Didn't *want* to stop it.

She wasn't sure which of them moved first, but the next thing she knew her arms were round his neck, his arms had tightened around her waist, and he was kissing her, his mouth sweet and gentle, offering temptation as well as comfort.

How could she resist letting him deepen the kiss?

Desire and need swept through her, pushing away the last vestiges of her common sense. The only thing that made her stop kissing him back was when an impatient car driver leaned on their horn, and the harsh sound crashed into her head.

She pulled back and stared at him.

What the hell had she just done?

Colour slashed across his face. 'I'm sorry, Mandy. I shouldn't have done that.'

It was noble of him to take responsibility, but it wasn't fair. She was just as much to blame. 'It wasn't just you,' she said. She'd been with him all the way. It was the first time she'd been kissed since she didn't know when, and it had put her into a total spin.

'I—look, I don't do relationships,' he said. 'It's complicated. But I don't. And that's not me trying to tell you in a nice way that I don't find you attractive, because actually I do. But that's exactly why I can't…' He closed his eyes briefly. 'Listen to me. Incoherence city. Sorry. I'm not usually this hopeless, this inarticulate. I don't kiss women at random. I…' He stared at her, as if he couldn't find the words to explain.

The words were jumbled in her head, too, but

she made the effort. 'Me, neither. I don't kiss men at random, I mean.'

'Mandy. I like you. A lot,' he emphasised. 'But all I can offer you is friendship.'

'Snap,' she said. 'I don't have time in my life for dating.' She didn't try to tell him that it wasn't her way of saying no gently, because it wasn't: and she was all too aware of how easy it would be to say that it didn't matter—that they were both middle-aged and single and they *could* do this, if they wanted. How easy it would be to slide her hands into his hair again and draw his head back down to hers. To touch her lips to his, offering and teasing and cajoling. To forget the world around them, the traffic and the people and the noise, and let herself drown in his kiss.

Though the sensible side of her knew that doing that would make life way too complicated. Daniel was her new job-share. She'd been working at the London Victoria for a week. It would be utterly insane to let anything more than friendship happen between them and risk making things awkward on the ward or in their shared office.

'So we're all right, you and me?' he checked.

She nodded. 'What happened just now was purely for comfort. For both of us. And it…' It was her turn to close her eyes for a moment. 'I'm shutting my mouth now, before I dig myself into a deeper hole.'

'I think we've both had the worst shift in months and we're feeling a bit wobbly right now,' he said. 'My recommendation for fixing that is—'

Another kiss, her libido supplied.

'—a good dose of carbs,' he said, and she was really glad that the words in her head hadn't burst out.

'My place is about ten minutes from here,' he continued. 'Or, since I don't have a clue what's in my fridge right now, we could walk up to King's Road—I know a good Italian trattoria there that does the most fabulous gnocchi.'

Even though a very big part of her was intrigued to see where Daniel lived, Mandy knew it would be a bad idea. They'd just agreed to be friends, but she had a nasty feeling that they were both still so wobbly that if they were alone it would be all too easy to start kissing again—and who knew where that might lead?

It would be much more sensible to stay in a public place. Talk themselves down from the edge of doing something risky.

'Gnocchi sounds fabulous,' she said. 'And we'll split the bill.'

'Fine by me,' he said. 'Because I like to think we'll become friends as well as colleagues.'

'I hope so, too,' she said. She liked what she'd seen of this man. The way he was with junior colleagues at work appealed to her; there was no boasting or trying to make himself look superior. He listened; he got them to talk and work things out for themselves but made it clear that he was there if they needed him. He was good with patients and with parents. And it was always good to have a friend.

They walked up to the restaurant. La Roma was pretty outside, with fairy lights and foliage decorating the enormous windows; inside, the floors were wooden and the pale terracotta walls were hung with photographs of iconic spots of Rome, from the Colosseum and the Pantheon to the Trevi Fountain. The small tables were covered with red-and-white-checked linen tablecloths; each had a small terracotta pot of herbs and a red candle set in an old raffia-covered Chianti bottle in the centre. And the scents from the kitchen were divine.

'What do you recommend?' she asked Daniel when the waiter had shown them to their seats, given them the menu, talked them through the specials on the chalkboard and brought them a jug of water when they admitted that neither of them was in the mood for a glass of wine.

'Everything I've ever eaten here has been excellent,' he said. 'But I'm having the gnocchi with gorgonzola sauce. Normally I try and have something different, but tonight I want the comfort of an old favourite.'

She scanned the menu. 'I'm tempted to join you, but then there's the mushroom risotto on the specials board. And I *love* risotto.' She blew out a breath. 'Though it feels *wrong*, enjoying choosing dinner after what happened today.'

He wrinkled his nose. 'I know what you mean—but today for me was a reminder that we never know what's going to happen in life. We should enjoy the little moments of joy when we can.'

'That's a good point,' she admitted.

Once they'd ordered, the waiter brought them a sharing board of olives, tiny arancini, marinated artichoke hearts and a creamy burrata along with some focaccia.

'The simple stuff's the best,' Daniel said. 'And they do it so well, here.'

'Do you come here often?' she asked.

'I normally bring the film crew here for dinner once a month, to say thank you,' he said. 'They're really good and make sure they don't intrude on the families or get in the way of the medics, so showing my appreciation is the least I can do. And I've brought my family here a few times.'

She noticed that he didn't mention girlfriends.

Not that she should be noticing that. Nothing was going to happen between them, and that flare of attraction she felt towards him needed to be buried. Pronto.

'What about you?' he asked. 'Do you eat out often?'

'With my best friend, after ballet class; sometimes with my mum and my sister; and I have dinner once a week with my daughter and son-in-law,' she said. 'Though more recently that's been at their place. Dev is an amazing cook. He's taught me a lot about Indian cuisine, and it's very far from chicken tikka masala.'

'It's nice that you're close to your family,' he said.

'I've been really lucky,' she said. 'When Gemma was small, I could never have managed without Mum and Dad and my big sister, Jen. You know what it's like as a junior doctor.'

'Long hours, being on call and never having enough sleep,' Daniel agreed. 'Your ex didn't help?'

She might as well tell him the truth. Particularly as it would be a useful barrier between them. 'My ex has never been part of Gemma's life,' she said. 'I didn't find out I was pregnant until after I'd filed for divorce. I did tell him about her existence, because I felt it would've been wrong not to tell him, but he made it clear he wasn't interested in being a dad, so if I kept her I'd be on my own. And that's how it's been ever since.' She sighed. 'Sometimes I feel guilty and think I should've found someone who would've made a good dad for Gemma. But I couldn't face dating again.'

Because she'd loved her ex that much? Daniel wondered. Then again, she'd just said she'd been the one to file for divorce. Not that he was going to ask her why; it was none of his business, and he didn't want to trample over old scars. 'I'm not sure that potentially being a good dad is enough of a reason to marry someone,' he said instead. 'I think you should marry someone because you want to spend your life with them.'

'That's what I thought I'd done,' she said. 'Laurence was charming, good company and I thought he was perfect. I met him at a party, fell for him like a ton of bricks, and six months later we were married. And I really thought everything was fine—until I came home sick from a night shift to find someone else in our bed with him.'

He winced. 'I'm sorry. That must've been a shock.'

She nodded. 'And then I found out she wasn't the first.' She shrugged. 'I guess not everyone can cope with a junior doctor's shifts. He got fed up with me not wanting to go to a party with him because I was on call or on nights, or being too tired to do anything after a long shift, or the fact I was still studying as well as working.'

'Plus, if you're not a medic, if you go to any social event you'll feel left out because everyone's talking about the hospital or gossiping about people you've never met,' Daniel said.

'That,' she said, 'sounds personal.'

'Yeah. My marriage didn't survive my houseman years—and it was my fault. I let the gap grow between us.' Which was only part of the truth. The rest of it was much more shameful.

'It takes two to break a marriage,' she said. 'In my case, Laurence decided to fill the gap with someone else.'

'I'm sorry he hurt you,' Daniel said. 'He was an idiot.' And now he knew he had to tell her the truth about his own marriage. OK, so it risked souring things between them, but at least it would remove some of the temptation if she knew the worst of him. Because, right now, he was looking at the curve of her mouth, remembering how well that curve had fitted to his own mouth, and wondering when he could kiss her again…

He took a deep breath. 'And I can say that because I made the same mistake.'

'Your ex cheated on you?'

He shook his head. 'I'm ashamed to say that I was the one who cheated. Things were getting rocky between us. We were both working long hours and getting snappy with each other—and then I met someone at work. Leila was three or four years older than me. Bright, sparkly, enormous fun. Everything I wanted—and I fell head over heels for her.' Exactly the same excuse his own father had used when Daniel, aged fifteen, had asked him why he'd cheated on Daniel's mother. Keith Monroe had blustered that he'd simply fallen head over heels in love with someone else. But then it had happened again. And again. When Daniel learned that the first affair he'd known about had been very far from the first one, he'd realised that his father was a serial cheat and a pathological liar, and he couldn't forgive Keith for it.

Daniel been so determined not to behave like his father did, especially as everyone said he was Keith's mini-me. He resembled his father in looks, and there wasn't much he could do about that; but he didn't want to be like his father in any other way. Maybe it was part of the reason he'd married Roxy so young; he'd wanted to prove to himself that he could offer his partner stability. That he could have a long-lasting, happy marriage.

Except it turned out that he really was a carbon copy of his father, letting himself fall for someone else when he was supposed to be committed to his wife. And that had horrified him. He didn't want to be 'all boys together' with his father, focusing on the thrill of the chase and not caring how he hurt his partner.

The night he'd split up with Roxy and Leila had responded by dumping him, he'd vowed to keep all relationships light, in future. Never again would he take the risk of repeating his mistake and hurting somebody else.

'I left my wife for Leila,' he said. 'It was the most stupid thing I'd ever done.' He'd been shocked to discover that Leila was a player; she'd seen her fling with him as nothing more than a bit of fun, and had been horrified to find out that his own intentions were serious. He'd wrecked his marriage for nothing, devastating both Roxy and himself—and it wasn't fixable. 'I bitterly regret the hurt I caused my ex.'

'You had an affair,' she said, her voice cool.

The collar on Daniel's shirt suddenly felt too tight. He'd wanted to put a barrier between them, show Mandy that he was the worst possible person she could think of falling for—she'd been cheated on, and he was a proven cheat. Unreliable. Though, at the same time, he didn't want her to despise him. Because he *wasn't* his father. 'I was very, very stupid and very, very wrong.'

He sighed. 'There are no excuses. Roxy and I met in the first week of university; we were inseparable as students and we got married the week after I graduated.' Maybe because he'd been so desperate to prove to himself that he could have a good, stable marriage. 'Looking back, we were probably too young to settle down, and we definitely didn't realise what kind of strain a junior doctor's hours can put on a relationship. But none of it was Roxy's fault.'

Mandy was silent for so long that Daniel started to wonder if she was going to get up and leave.

Then she looked at him. 'At least you're shouldering the blame instead of trying to dump it on your wife.'

'Of course I'm not going to try to blame her. She didn't do anything wrong. I regret what I did. *Not* because I got caught,' he emphasised, 'but because I hurt her and she didn't deserve that.'

'And you didn't stay with the woman you had the affair with?'

That stung, but he knew he deserved the question. 'I planned to, but she dumped me. It turned out that half my attraction for her was that I was involved with someone else—which made me forbidden fruit. As soon as I left Roxy and asked Leila to make it serious, she broke up with me.'

'So she didn't actually care about you?'

'No.' He grimaced. 'And I was young and naive enough not to see it in the first place. I got burned. But I know I hurt Roxy even more, so I'm not looking for sympathy. It was my own fault.'

Her brown eyes narrowed as she assessed him. 'That's honest,' she said.

'And I've been honest ever since,' he said. 'It's why I don't do serious relationships. I make it clear to anyone who dates me that it's going to be just for fun, just for now, and I'm not looking for forever.'

'I don't do relationships, either,' she said. 'Not because I'm still in love with Laurence, because I'm not. I just don't have the time or the space in my life for anything else.' She took a deep breath and gave him a wry smile. 'And, if I'm being honest, I guess it's a little hard to trust again after that...'

Which told Daniel exactly where he stood with her; and he definitely needed to damp down the attraction he felt towards her, because it most certainly wasn't going to be reciprocated. Once bitten, definitely twice shy.

'Did you try to get back together with Roxy, when it all went sour with Leila?' she asked.

'No. I could hardly go running back to her

and tell her I'd made a mistake. I decided to give us both a bit of time to get over the bitterness, and then see if there was a way we could move forward. But I left it too long, because when we talked she told me she'd met someone else at work,' he said. 'She said she thought we'd got together too young and we'd started growing apart. She probably had a point. But that still doesn't excuse what I did. I'd made a commitment, and I should've just pushed through the difficult stuff and stuck by her. Instead, I let myself get distracted by Leila. I took the easy option—and it was wrong.'

'Thank you for being open with me,' she said. 'And I'd like to assure you that I won't be gossiping about anything you just told me.'

'Thank you. I won't be gossiping about you, either,' he said. 'And I'd like to assure you that my past idiocy in my private life doesn't apply to my work. Ever.'

'I've already seen that for myself,' she said. 'I'm pretty sure we'll rub along OK together in the job.'

He didn't dare ask her about whether they'd still become friends, now. He'd probably derailed that, too, with his confession. And he was seriously relieved when their food arrived. If he filled his mouth with carbs, maybe it would stop him saying something else he'd regret later.

* * *

In some ways, Mandy wasn't surprised by what Daniel had just confessed. He was even more charming than Laurence, and she'd learned the hard way that charming men were unreliable.

In other ways, she was shocked. The kind, caring man she'd been working with at the hospital had too big a heart to be unfaithful, surely?

Then again, his affair had happened half a lifetime ago. She wasn't the same now as she'd been in her twenties; doubtless Daniel had changed over the years, too. And it sounded as if he'd been vulnerable at the time, struggling with his marriage and his job, and he'd fallen for someone who'd treated him just as badly as Laurence had treated her. He'd told her that he didn't date; clearly the fallout from his marriage ending had made him avoid relationships as much as she had.

Daniel was probably the worst person she could ever let herself fall for.

It would be much more sensible for them to stick to being colleagues, maybe friends.

'Is your risotto all right?' he asked.

'Lovely, thank you.' She winced, hearing how stilted her words sounded. It wasn't her place to judge his past. 'It's actually delicious. Would you like to try some?'

Colour rose in his face again. Not surprising,

because sharing a taste of your meal was something you'd do with a lover. She should've chosen her words more carefully, or picked some anodyne topic of conversation. The weather, holidays, work… Where was easy small talk, when you needed it?

'Thanks for the offer, but I'm happy to stick with my pasta. Which you're welcome to try,' he added hastily.

'You're finding this as awkward as I am, aren't you?' she asked.

'Yes.' He sighed. 'This evening was meant to be a walk to clear my head and having dinner with a colleague who'd shared my rough day. A chance to decompress a bit. And what do I do? I kiss you stupid, I'm nosey about your ex, and I tell you I'm basically your worst nightmare.'

'Agreed. Though, actually, I think I might've kissed you, first,' she said. 'And I was the one who brought up my ex.'

'So where do we go from here?' he asked.

'I think,' she said, 'we muddle through and try to be kind to each other. And maybe avoid being in a situation where we might end up…well, too close to each other,' she added.

'Work's fine. We're not going to do anything stupid in our office or on the ward, not when we both know what a hospital grapevine can be like,' Daniel said. 'But outside—agreed. Only public places. If we go for a walk together, we'll make sure there are no secluded bits.'

'Technically, the Chelsea embankment doesn't count as secluded,' she pointed out. And still they'd ended up kissing, in full view of anyone passing by.

'True.' He raised an eyebrow. 'I guess we just have to keep reminding each other to be sensible.'

'Works for me,' she said, raising her glass of water. 'Friends.'

'Friends,' he said, chinking his glass against hers.

They managed to split the dessert sharing board of orange polenta cake, tiramisu and an amazing apple tart served with cinnamon cream without their fingers accidentally brushing.

'It's probably not a good idea to invite you back for coffee,' he said.

'Definitely,' she agreed.

'Can I call you a cab? The nearest Tube is Sloane Square, and that's a ten-minute walk. In the rain.'

'My coat has a hood,' she said. 'I'm fine getting the Tube—I don't even have to change lines from Sloane Square to get to King's Cross. And you don't need to walk me to the station, either.'

'My mother would say otherwise—and so would yours, I bet,' he said.

'Our mothers are from a different generation,'

she retorted. 'If you walk me to the station, I'll be tempted to give you a hug goodbye. And you know what our last hug led to.'

'That was before we agreed to keep things platonic,' he argued.

'Even so,' she said firmly. 'We're splitting the bill, walking in separate directions, and we'll see each other tomorrow at the hospital.'

'And now I know,' he said, 'you're not going to be a pushover as joint Head of Paediatrics. You'll give the suits as good as you get.'

'Better,' she said, 'because nobody's getting away with being a cheapskate with our ward.'

They split the bill, said goodbye in the middle of the restaurant, and after he held the door for her they walked in opposite directions.

Part of Mandy liked the fact Daniel had wanted to walk her to the station. But she knew they'd made the right decision. If he'd walked with her, it would've been too easy for their hands to brush, then cling together—and this time it wouldn't have been merely for comfort. Both of them would've thought about that kiss. Both of them would've acted on that kiss. And it would all end up in an awkward, difficult mess.

All she had to do now was wipe that kiss from her memory.

Though her mouth would have to stop tingling, first…

CHAPTER FIVE

DANIEL COULDN'T GET that kiss out of his head. The softness of Mandy's mouth. The way it had fitted so perfectly against his. The feel of her hands tangling in his hair.

A cold shower didn't help much.

Neither did counting backwards from five hundred in seventeens.

Or the cryptic crossword.

Or a run before work, on Tuesday morning.

Or the triple-strength coffee he made in the staff kitchen on the way to his desk.

All he could think about was her. What the hell was he going to do about this?

He'd read an article about wearing an elastic band around your wrist and pinging it when you needed to distract yourself from thinking something. Maybe that would work. Except of course there wasn't an elastic band to be found anywhere in his desk.

Focus, Daniel, he told himself grimly.

This was a work environment, not a place to

let his mind roam free. He was going to concentrate on the paperwork he'd come in early to finish. And he managed it. He even filed some of it.

But then Mandy turned up. Bringing coffee—and an almond croissant.

'Peace offering,' she said. 'And because you're doing the debrief this morning. You need carbs before that.'

'That's kind,' he said, touched. 'I appreciate this. Very much.'

'You're welcome.' She lifted one shoulder in a shrug. 'There's a nice bakery between my flat and the station, and they open early.'

And she'd thought of him. Thought of the horrible morning he had ahead, and bought something to bolster him. It warmed him all the way through.

Maybe they could be friends, after all. Just as long as he managed to stop himself thinking about kissing her again.

He wished he'd thought of buying biscuits for the team at the debrief. As it was, the best he could do was be open with his team. 'We all did our best, yesterday. Nobody could've done more for little Aarya, and nobody's to blame for her death,' he said. 'How are you all doing, this morning?'

'Grim,' Khaj said. 'We don't have many deaths on this ward. And they hurt.'

'I know they do,' he said gently. 'We wouldn't be any good as medics if we didn't feel the losses. But I don't want you to feel you have to carry on as if nothing had happened, see your next patient and smile.'

'To be fair, we *do* have to see our next patients and smile,' Ginny, one of the junior doctors, said. 'We can't stop treating people.'

'But we don't have to carry on as if nothing had happened. It's all right to take a moment. To acknowledge how you're feeling,' he said. 'I don't want any of you to feel you're burning out. So if you need to talk to someone after we lose a patient—whether it's me, Mandy or a counsellor—that's fine. It's a sign of strength, not weakness, to recognise you need help and to ask for it.'

'The palliative care team at my old hospital used to hold weekly meetings, and someone would read a poem or a multi-faith prayer,' Mandy said. 'They said it helped. We were going to start trialling that with my team.'

'It's an interesting idea,' Daniel said. 'Can you all have a think about whether you'd like to do something like that? We could probably manage it on Wednesday mornings when Mandy isn't up to her neck in students and I'm not filming.'

'Actually, if we do this, it'd be good to include the students,' Mandy said. 'We should teach them about self-care and show them how to cope with the rough bits of the job.'

'Agreed,' Khaj said. 'And maybe we can take it in turns to bring in cake or what have you.'

Daniel chuckled. 'No arguments from me on that one.' He paused. 'While we're here, I'd like to review our procedures for infant cardiac arrests and check we're all on the same page. And if anyone has any questions, I'm listening.'

After the debrief, Daniel checked in on baby Noah. Lucy Carmichael was sitting with him, reading him a story.

'How are you doing?' he asked.

'Getting there,' she said. 'Everyone's been so kind. And we're starting to see improvements. Mo says we can try taking him off assisted breathing, at the end of the week.'

'That's good,' Daniel said. 'Though if it turns out he's not ready for it yet, try not to worry. These things take time, and we can't always predict them.'

'All right,' she said.

'Given that he's improving,' Daniel said, 'would you and Rob consider letting Noah be one of our case studies on the *London Victoria Children's Ward* documentary?'

Her eyes widened. 'He'd be on TV?'

'Only with your permission, and there's absolutely no pressure. It won't make any difference to the care he receives whether you say yes or no. Talk it over with Rob.'

'I guess it'd be a warning about what could happen if a baby's given honey,' Lucy said. 'And it might get the message across to people who haven't thought about it before—or those who take the attitude that it didn't hurt them or their own kids.'

'It might,' Daniel agreed. 'And it'd be nice to show other parts of the hospital working as a team, bits that patients and visitors never really see. I'd love the chance to bring in the pharmacy team. But, as I said, there's no pressure. Talk to Rob, and if you're both interested then come and ask me any questions you might have. I can also put you in touch with other parents who've been part of the series, to give you a better idea about what to expect.'

'I will,' Lucy said.

On Wednesday afternoon, Daniel caught up with Mandy. 'Now Noah's recovering, the Carmichaels have given me permission to use him as a case study on the show. As you're the one who worked out what was wrong, would you like to be part of it?'

She looked surprised. 'Me, on TV?'

'If you'd rather not be on camera,' he said, 'I'll still make sure you get the credit you deserve and I'll explain how you worked it out. Have a think about it. If you'd like to see how we film a case, I've got Matthew Field in tomorrow—he's ten and he's in for his last surgery for Shone's syndrome.'

'Shone's—that's where the heart structures don't form properly on the left, isn't it?' Mandy asked.

'Yes—three out of the eight possible problems, in Matty's case. He's had quite a few surgeries over the years. We're filming him and his mum in the morning. If you sit in on it, you can meet the crew and see how we work. Matty's mum, Theresa, is getting to be quite an old hand at this now.'

'Do I need to keep out of the office on Thursdays and Fridays when you're filming?' she asked.

'Not very much,' he said. 'Most of what we do is a fly-on-the-wall approach, so we'll be in the consulting rooms, operating theatres and on the ward. If we do need to use the office, I'll stick a note on the door saying how long we'll be.'

'This is all really interesting,' Mandy said. 'I've spoken to journalists before, back at Muswell Hill, but I've never done anything with TV broadcasting.'

'It's not as glamorous as you might think,' he warned. 'We're a small team, and there's a lot of repetition to make sure we get the footage we need. Some of the time Shalmi will film me nodding my head, so if we have to cut bits we have some visuals to help with continuity.'

'OK. What time do you need me in?'

'We start filming at ten,' he said. 'So, after ward rounds works for me.'

'Got it,' she said.

On Thursday morning, after she'd finished ward rounds, Mandy went into the office to meet Daniel's film crew.

'Everyone, this is Mandy, who's the joint Head of Paediatrics with me,' Daniel said. 'Mandy, this is Shalmi, our camerawoman; Carey, who's in charge of light and sound; and Keisha, our producer.'

'Otherwise known as the person who sorts the schedules, trouble-shoots and drives everyone mad bossing them about,' Keisha said with a smile. 'Dan tells me you've agreed to be filmed as part of Noah's story—you're the one who worked out what was wrong with him.'

'It was a hunch,' Mandy said.

'A good one, and you're the only one who suggested it,' Daniel reminded her. 'Mandy, this is Theresa Field, Matthew's mum; and Matty, who's having his final surgery later this morning. We'd hoped to do it before he started high school, but now he gets to miss half a term of football.'

'I don't mind,' Matty said with a grin. 'Cricket's way better than football anyway, and I'll be well again before the cricket season starts.'

'Nice to meet you, Theresa and Matty,' Mandy said, shaking their hands in turn. 'I'm one of the doctors on the ward, so I'll probably see you on ward rounds. I teach students on Mondays and Tuesdays. Thank you for letting me sit in on your interview.'

'No problem,' Theresa said. 'We're quite used to talking to the cameras, now.'

'As last year, we'll be cutting your story with the photographs you lent us and some footage of similar operations,' Keisha said, 'to show Matty's journey so far.'

Shalmi took some test shots, Carey adjusted the lighting and then Daniel started talking to Theresa, who explained her son's story.

'When Matty was born, he struggled with breathing, and the doctor told us he had critical aortic stenosis—that meant his blood couldn't flow properly through his heart. The next day, they gave him keyhole surgery and put a balloon into the valve so they could open it. He recovered well, but then he went into heart failure. He was taken to Intensive Care and put on life support.' Theresa swallowed hard. 'Even now, remembering how tiny he was, how sick he was and how scared we were makes me well up. But the staff were brilliant. They saved his life. Matty had open heart surgery to repair the valve, and five months later they created a new circuit in his heart so it could pump enough blood around his body.'

'I was in hospital quite a lot over the next few years,' Matty said, 'but Mum and Dad could stay in a flat just round the corner so they could be with me, and I did a lot of my lessons here. Later today I'm going to have open heart surgery again, which will help my circulation, and we hope it'll be the last big operation I need. I know I'm never going to be able to play really fast sports or climb a mountain, because I get out of puff, but I've joined my local cricket team.' His smile broadened. 'One day, I want to play for England as a really ace bowler, but for now I'm happy to play for the village.'

'And I'm looking forward to cheering our Matty as he takes out all the opposition's wickets,' Daniel added.

Keisha reviewed the footage and got Theresa and Matty to repeat a couple of bits, and add in some different information, and then it was done.

'Well done, Team Field,' Daniel said. 'Khaj is

going to settle you in on the ward, Matty, and the surgeon will be along to see you shortly.'

'Good,' Matty said, and his stomach growled. 'I'm *starving*. The worst bit of having an operation is not being allowed to have breakfast!'

'Oh, wait—I want that,' Keisha said.

'Don't tell me—smile and repeat it?' Matty teased, clearly used to the filming routine.

'If you can make your stomach growl again, that would be cool,' Keisha said, 'but a smile will do.'

Matty duly repeated his comment for the camera.

'Do either of you have any questions for me?' Daniel asked Theresa and Matty.

'No—I think my last questions are for the surgeon,' Theresa said.

'Which I'll be filming,' Shalmi said.

Once Khaj had collected Matty, it was Mandy's turn to speak to camera, explaining how baby Noah's symptoms hadn't made any sense until she remembered a case her friend had come across on secondment in America, and they'd realised that the baby had infant botulism.

'That was good,' Keisha said. 'I'm going to make you redo all that from a slightly different angle—not because you got anything wrong, but because I want to cover several angles. And

I might need you again later, depending on how it looks when we cut everything together.'

'Sure,' Mandy said.

She was busy on the ward and in the office for the rest of the day, and on Friday morning she was filmed in their shared office for a few last tweaks.

'Thank you for all your help,' Daniel said. 'I think our viewers are going to find this all really interesting.'

'I agree,' she said. 'And it's really good to see how things have changed for Matty's family—from all the worry of his first couple of days through to the well-balanced pre-teen he is now.'

Later that afternoon, Mandy was just finishing her last bit of admin when Daniel came back into the office and smiled at her. 'Have fun at ballet tonight.'

'Thank you. I will.'

She noticed a tide of colour sweep into his face and wondered what had caused it. She knew she ought to act as if she hadn't noticed, but the question burst out of her anyway. 'Dan? What is it?'

He groaned. 'God. I'm blushing, aren't I? My face feels hot.'

She nodded, and he closed his eyes. 'Sorry. Just pretend I look normal.'

But he didn't. And, even though part of her

knew this would be dangerous, she wanted to know what was in his head. 'Dan,' she said softly. 'Talk to me.'

He opened his eyes again and looked at her. 'You want the truth? All right. I can't get you out of my head, Mandy. I haven't been able to stop thinking about you since Monday night. And I shouldn't have mentioned ballet, because right now I'm imagining you in a sparkly leotard and a tutu, pirouetting towards me at the end of the Sugar Plum Fairy solo, and ending up in my arms.'

And now the picture was in her head, too. Along with the music.

'I'm not a proper ballerina, Dan. I don't wear pointe shoes, just normal soft ballet shoes. It's a beginner class for older adults and the most we do is demi-pointe—tiptoes,' she said.

'That doesn't help,' he said. 'Actually, if anything, you've just made it worse. Because now in my head you're barefoot on the sand, dancing towards me in a swishy skirt. Still to the Sugar Plum Fairy music, because that's my favourite bit of the entire ballet.' He dragged in a breath. 'Ignore me. I'll get my common sense back. I'll have lots of cold showers and keep my distance.'

'What if you didn't have to?' The words came out before she could stop them, and suddenly there wasn't any air in the room.

He took his glasses off and sat down at his desk, opposite hers. His gaze was intense. 'I don't do relationships, Mandy.'

'And you've been honest about the reason for that. So I know you're not going to cheat on me,' she said.

'I'm really not a good bet. Mercurial, my mother calls me, but it's not...' He gave an odd smile. 'Mercutio, maybe. The annoying friend who's always the joker, always lightening the mood, shallow as a puddle. We've all got one in our lives. Except I think I'm the Mercutio in everyone's life. Ballet Mercutio, that is, not Shakespeare Mercutio. I'm about fun, not fighting.'

'That's a good life skill,' she said softly, 'being able to lighten someone's mood. Talk them out of a dark space. Not many people are good at it. Don't do yourself down.'

'I never, ever let myself feel like this,' he said. 'Not about anyone. But I can't stop thinking about you.'

'Same here,' she said. 'I don't have time in my life for a relationship. I don't want to date anyone. But when we kissed...' She bit her lip. 'Dan, we can't talk about this here. Not when someone might walk in and hear us.'

'How about tonight?' he asked. 'After your class?'

'I'm having dinner with Linda, then,' she said.

'Though I could ask her to cancel.' Her best friend would understand. More than understand. Linda would probably tell her to skip the class, dance for him instead, and have a mad, crazy fling—that it would do her good.

'You have a busy life. A life you love,' he said softly. 'I'm not going to disrupt that.'

Though she had the nasty feeling that he really could. If she let him close, Daniel could disrupt *everything*.

She could make herself resist the temptation. Eventually the attraction would die down.

Except…

Since that kiss, she didn't want to resist any more. Which was exhilarating and terrifying in equal measures.

'How about tomorrow?' he suggested. 'We'll do this the practical way. Talk. Over lunch.'

'In a public place,' she said. Where they'd have to contain themselves.

'That would be prudent,' he said. 'Except I don't want to be sensible. If I'm going to have lunch with you, I want to cook for you.' He gave another of those odd, self-deprecating smiles. 'That's Dan the show-off talking. TV Dan. Shallow. Dr TWC.'

'I don't think you're shallow,' she said. 'I think you like everyone to believe you are, but you're not. You just don't let people close enough to see who you really are.'

'You,' he said, 'are terrifying.'

'So,' she whispered, 'are you.'

'I'm not scary. Not in the slightest,' he protested. 'Mercutio Dan, that's me. Dan of the terrible jokes.'

Daniel whose kiss made her feel as if the world had melted away. Not that she was going to say that out loud. Not here, at least, because the last thing either of them needed was to be the hottest gossip on the hospital grapevine. 'Tomorrow,' she said. 'Text me your address. And I'll bring pudding.'

At ballet class, as always, Mandy had to concentrate on what her arms and legs were doing, and there wasn't space to think about Daniel and wonder if she'd temporarily taken leave of her senses.

Afterwards, she went for dinner with her best friend at a little bistro round the corner from the dance school, and confessed all. 'The thing is, Lin,' she said, 'I can't get him out of my head, and he can't get me out of his. I've agreed to have lunch with him tomorrow. We're going to talk it through.'

'Which sounds perfectly rational,' Linda said.

Mandy wrinkled her nose. 'It would be, if we were going to be in a public place. But he's cooking for me. At his house. And…' She shook her head. 'Maybe I was temporarily insane to agree to it. We kissed in the middle of the street. What's going to happen in a private space?' She bit her lip. 'Would I be wiser to call the whole thing off?'

'If you call it off,' Linda pointed out, 'you're going to spend the entire weekend brooding about it and wishing you'd been braver.'

'If I go… What if something happens?'

Linda sang a snatch of The Clash's 'Should I Stay or Should I Go' and spread her hands.

'That's just it,' Mandy said ruefully. 'I think we're both scared of what could happen. Neither of us wants a serious relationship.'

'Not every guy's a Laurence,' Linda reminded her. 'There are good men out there who don't cheat.'

Mandy sighed. 'I'm not gossiping about him, because you're my best friend and I know you won't say a word to anyone else about this, but his marriage broke up because he was the one who cheated.'

Linda frowned. 'Hang on. I thought he was single?'

'He is. This all happened half a lifetime ago,' Mandy said. 'He's had a three-dates-and-it's-over policy since then, because he doesn't want to risk hurting anyone again.'

'I'm not making excuses for him, but half a lifetime ago we were all still very young and we didn't always make good choices,' Linda said. 'But if he's stuck to keeping every relationship short and sweet, since then—that's the opposite of what Laurence would do. Laurence is the sort who strings every relationship along until he thinks he can get a better offer.'

'I think Daniel's never been able to forgive himself for what he did,' Mandy said.

'In which case, he's definitely not going to hurt you. If he's got a three-date rule, you could have a three-date fling with him,' Linda suggested.

'I could,' Mandy said. 'But what if we get to the end of date three and that's still not enough?'

'You're breaking your rules to have a fling with him in the first place, so he can meet you halfway and break his own rules to have a longer fling with you,' Linda said.

'Maybe. But what i—?'

'Mand, I love you dearly, but you're overthinking this,' Linda interrupted gently. 'You're both in your fifties. You're both perfectly capable of keeping your private life and your professional life separate. So just *do* it. Have the fling. Get it out of your systems. And then you can stay on friendly terms and it'll be fine at work.'

'It's that simple?' Mandy asked.

'It's that simple,' Linda said firmly.

Mandy's phone beeped in her bag.

'Check it,' Linda advised, 'or you'll be worrying it's Gemma and she's gone into labour really early.'

'She'd call me, not text, if there was a problem,' Mandy said.

'I know we normally try to avoid tech at the table, but I think you should at least look and see who it's from,' Linda said.

Mandy did so, and felt the colour flood into her face. 'It's Daniel. Giving me his address. Checking if there's anything I don't eat.' She smiled. 'He says he's making me *mezze*.'

'Let me get this straight. He's gorgeous, he respects the nursing team, he's good with the patients and their parents, he tells the kind of jokes you like *and* he can cook? Why on earth are you dithering about this?' Linda shook her head. 'Actually, I think you should've cancelled dinner with me tonight and gone to see him straight after class.'

'He likes ballet, too. He took his niece to see *The Nutcracker* when she was six.' Mandy thought of what he'd said in the office with the door shut, about her pirouetting towards him, and her skin heated even more.

'He sounds like a man worth breaking your

rules for,' Linda said. 'Give yourself permission to have that fling, Mand. Because I think you'll really regret it if you don't.'

CHAPTER SIX

HE AND MANDY were simply having lunch. Talking it through—no, talking themselves down from having a fling, Daniel reminded himself. Being sensible. So why did this feel like a date? And not like the 'have fun but keep them at an emotional distance' date he specialised in, but a proper 'let's take a chance and see where this takes us' kind of date?

He forced himself to focus on cooking. Mandy had texted him back last night to say that she ate practically anything but preferred to avoid red meat, so he'd put together a menu he hoped she'd like, given that she'd enjoyed their sharing board. He'd made a smoky aubergine dip, which was on the table along with a crisp green salad, a bowl of hummus, a bowl of large green Kalamata olives and a bowl of heritage tomatoes. In the oven, he had spinach and feta borek cooking, along with chicken mini fillets that he'd rubbed with sumac, pomegranate molasses and chilli flakes, and spiced roasted cauliflower. The tahini dip for the cauliflower was ready, along with a bowl of pomegranate seeds to sprinkle over it. The flatbread dough was proving and ready to cook on the griddle pan; and the house was tidy. There wasn't anything else he could do.

Mandy wasn't the sort who'd just not turn up at the last minute; he was pretty sure that if she'd changed her mind she would've texted him earlier. But Daniel still found himself feeling nervous, pacing the room and picking things up for no reason and putting them down.

Oh, for pity's sake. This was *lunch*.

But it felt like something else. Like the start of something that could change everything...

Mandy walked from Sloane Square Tube station, heading towards the Chelsea Physic Garden and checking on her phone app that she was going in the right direction. Finally, she turned onto Daniel's street and checked the house numbers as she walked along. The road had several blocks of three-storey Georgian townhouses with a white stucco ground floor and yellow London brick for the upper storeys; the houses all had beautiful big sash windows and tall chimney pots in a row. The doors were painted a glossy black and had a brass door knocker, letter box and doorknob; there was an old-fashioned bell press at the side of the door, with an old-fashioned lantern light above it which matched the equally old-fashioned lantern-style streetlights.

Most of the townhouses had a small square front garden with wrought iron railings, which was laid to stone flags and contained lots of terracotta pots filled with pruned rose bushes and shrubs. There wasn't much colour at this time of year, but no doubt the street looked incredibly pretty in summer.

At last she came to Daniel's front door and took a deep breath. This was it. Her heart was beating a mad tattoo; it felt like being a teenager on a first date with a boy she'd liked from afar all year.

Her best friend's words echoed in her head: *'He sounds like a man worth breaking your rules for. Give yourself permission to have that fling, Mand. Because I think you'll really regret it if you don't.'*

Maybe.

Maybe not.

But there was only one way to find out.

She took a deep breath, raised the knocker—this was it, no going back—and rapped three times.

A few moments later, Daniel arrived at the door. He was dressed casually in faded jeans and a plain white shirt, and looked ridiculously sexy.

'Hi.' He smiled at her and her heart felt as if it had done an anatomically impossible backflip.

'Hi. You said you were doing *mezze*, so I thought about cheating massively and bringing a pot of Greek yogurt and fresh fruit for pudding,' she said, 'but I know you're a cake fiend. So I hope you like this.' She handed him the tote bag containing a cake tin.

'Thank you,' he said. 'I'm sure I will.'

'It's *karythopita*—a Greek spiced walnut cake. I made one for my sister and my mum, too.' And now she was gabbling.

Shut up, Mandy, she told herself silently.

'May I?' He opened the lid of the cake tin, took a sniff and grinned. 'That smells glorious. I'm tempted to skip the entire main course and just scoff this.'

His enthusiasm made her smile. 'You're an adult,' she said. 'You can do whatever you choose. Pudding instead of mains, cake for breakfast…'

'I like the way you're thinking, but my sister and my mum would tell you not to encourage me,' he said with a smile. 'Come in. Let me take your coat and get you a drink.'

'I'm on call,' she reminded him, 'so I need to stick to soft drinks.'

'I thought you might say that,' he said, 'so I made a jug of alcohol-free pomegranate mojito—it's my sister-in-law Sasha's recipe.' He closed the door behind them, took her coat and hung it on the bentwood stand in the entrance hall. 'Righty. Come through. The loo's there, under the stairs, if you need it.'

'Should I take my shoes off?' she asked.

'No, you're fine,' he said with a smile.

The whole of the ground floor seemed to be one large reception room; the flooring was all beautiful light parquet, and the walls were painted a pale sage green that went with the Georgian high ceilings and made the room feel light. There was a comfortable-looking chester-field-style sofa upholstered in sage green, with two armchairs opposite it, and a coffee table on the Persian rug in between them. The TV was set above the fireplace; there were shelves of books that she itched to browse through, wondering what kind of thing he read.

Once past the stairs and the cloakroom, the room opened out further with the kitchen running along one wall; the cabinets and worktops were cream and of a plain design that complemented the style of the house. There was a dining table big enough for eight on the other side of the room set underneath a glass roof, leading to French doors that looked out onto a small and very neat courtyard garden. Next to the door were a standard lamp shaped like a globe, and a zinc tub containing a large, variegated rubber plant. It was incredibly stylish, yet at the same time it felt warm and welcoming.

Daniel took a jug from the fridge and poured them both a glass of pomegranate mojito. 'The stuff in the oven is almost ready; I just need to cook the flatbreads on the griddle pan, which will take about two minutes.'

'Is there anything I can do to help?' she asked.

'Sit and chat to me.' He indicated the table, which had an array of delicious-looking mezze set out on it, and two places were set opposite each other at the end nearest the garden.

'This is delicious,' she said after a sip of her mojito. 'Refreshing and not too sweet.'

'Perfect for summer barbecues,' he said. 'But it's also nice in winter. It reminds me of the sunshine.'

'Your house is lovely,' she said.

'Thank you. It's the light that made me fall in love with it.' He smiled. 'The previous owner used some of the garden to make the kitchen wider, adding the glass roof and the glass wall, so this end is a kind of a kitchen-cum-conservatory-cum-garden-room, and it's all full of light. I love it when the family comes over and we all sit round the table and talk; then after dinner we can just leave everything where it is and go and collapse on the sofas and carry on talking.'

A sound system somewhere was playing piano music.

'Is this OK or would you prefer me to change it?' he asked.

'It's lovely—Einaudi, isn't it?'

'Yes. I find it good to chill to.' He raised his eyebrows. 'Though I do have a fairly broad taste. Everything from my big brother's old punk rock records through to Abba from when Daisy was a tot and insisted on playing "Dancing Queen" on repeat. And by "repeat", I mean for a good ten or eleven times in a row, until we could talk her into letting us play something else.'

He sounded like a completely devoted uncle; he would've made a good father, too, Mandy thought. Very unlike Gemma's own father.

She watched him deftly cook the flatbreads and transfer them from the griddle pan to a serving dish; then he served up the rest of the meal.

'I admit to buying the hummus. Whatever I do, I can never get the texture right, and there's a good deli round the corner—the olives come from there, too,' he said. 'But I made everything else.'

'It all looks fabulous,' she said. When she'd helped herself to a little of everything and tried it, she added, 'And it tastes even better.'

'Thank you. I enjoy cooking,' he said.

'Me, too,' she said.

They kept the conversation light until they'd finished lunch, he'd eaten two slices of cake and he'd made coffee.

'Can I at least wash up?' Mandy asked.

'That's what the dishwasher is for,' he said.

'No more excuses for avoiding *that* conversation, then,' she said.

'No. And you're right—we need to face it head on instead of skirting around it.' He looked at her. 'I still can't stop thinking about you.'

'Snap.' She paused. 'I hope you don't mind— I talked about the situation with my best friend, last night. Linda's known me since our first day at uni, and I trust her completely. She won't gossip or run to the tabloids about you.'

'I envy you,' he said. 'I can talk to my best friend about work and money and practical stuff, but neither of us would know where to start about emotional stuff. We'd both be squirming.'

'That's pretty standard for our generation,' she said. 'I think the next one down from us has more of a clue.'

'I hope so.' He paused. 'What's her verdict?'

'I have a no-date rule. You have a three-date rule. Linda thinks we're old enough to be able to separate work and…other stuff.'

'So we break the rules and see what happens?'

Her mouth was too dry to let her speak, so she nodded.

'Interesting,' he said. 'I assume, since you knew her from your student days, she knew your ex.'

'She was one of my bridesmaids. And she never liked Laurence,' Mandy admitted. 'She said he was vain.'

Daniel gave a bark of laughter. 'And a TV doc isn't vain, by definition?'

'You're not vain,' Mandy said. 'Not with that hair.'

'Believe me, I'm vain. I changed my outfit twice before you got here,' he confessed. 'Jeans and a T-shirt looked too casual and I didn't want you thinking I couldn't be bothered to make an effort. A proper shirt and trousers looked too much like a work outfit and as if I was trying to keep you at a professional distance.' He indicated his jeans and shirt. 'This was a compromise.'

He'd changed twice, for her? She couldn't help smiling. 'You know what? Me, too. A dress felt like overkill, not a relaxed Saturday lunch between friends. My black trousers are smart, but I looked as if I was about to go into work—as you say, putting a professional distance between us.' She indicated her top. 'This made my trousers feel a bit less formal. But, as you say, still making a bit of an effort.'

'That floaty top is really pretty,' he said. 'It suits you.'

'Thank you. And you look sexy as hell.' She closed her eyes. 'Uh. What is it about you that makes me blurt out whatever's in my head instead of filtering it like a sensible person would?'

'The same thing about you that makes me blush all the time, I think,' Daniel said. 'So what do we do now? Follow your best friend's advice?'

'A fling. We don't put an end date on it before it starts, but we keep it fun,' she said. 'So neither of us gets hurt.'

'That works for me,' he said.

'At work,' she said, 'we're colleagues. Friendly, but colleagues. Professional. And it stays that way when our fling ends.'

'Agreed,' he said. 'And outside work…'

They'd be lovers. A shiver went down her spine.

'It's been a long time, for me,' she whispered. 'I have no idea any more what you're supposed to do on a date.'

'I don't date anywhere near as much as the media likes to make out,' he said. 'And right at this moment I feel as clueless as a teenager.'

'Like standing on the edge of a cliff, knowing you're supposed to jump in but not sure if you can remember how to swim,' she said.

He pushed his chair back, walked round the

table to her, and held out his hand. 'Then let's jump. Together.'

She took his hand and let him draw her to her feet. The butterflies in her stomach were doing what felt like a stampede.

'Now what?' she asked shakily.

'Dance with me?' he asked. 'I'll change the music.'

He instructed the smart speaker to play 'Something' by George Harrison.

The perfect song, she thought.

'A pedant would point out that it's actually by The Beatles,' she said.

'Bring it on. I've got George Harrison's *Best Of* on vinyl upstairs, and this is the first track,' he retorted.

She laughed. 'I want to look through your vinyl. And your bookshelves.'

'Any time you like,' he said. 'But right now I want five minutes just to hold you in my arms and dance with you.'

Slow dancing on a Saturday afternoon in late autumn, when it was grey outside yet warm inside, felt perfect. Dancing cheek to cheek, because he'd stooped slightly to accommodate the fact she was shorter than he was, even with her shoes on. His hands settled round her waist, and hers were looped round his neck.

She closed her eyes, enjoying his nearness.

And slowly, as they swayed together, their faces turned slightly, so the corners of their mouths were touching. Turning further, so his lips were brushing against hers, making every nerve-end tingle. And then they were really kissing, holding each other close, lost in the magic of a kiss.

When he finally broke the kiss, she felt dazed. And no music at all was playing—the song had clearly ended and the sound system had paused.

'Um...' He stroked her face. 'Sorry.'

'No need to apologise. I think we're both on the same page,' she said lightly.

He gave her a wry smile. 'I might just have turned into a troglodyte, wanting to carry you up the stairs to my lair.'

She laughed. 'You don't need to carry me.' She paused. This was where she could leave—or she could stay. Adrenaline pulsed through her, and she decided to take the risk. 'You could always just show me where your lair is.'

'One problem,' he said, his expression suddenly serious. 'Unless you have a condom in your bag... I don't have any.'

She appreciated his concern—and the fact he'd been honest with her. So she could be honest, too. 'Do we need one?' she asked. 'I'm through the menopause so I can't get pregnant, and I haven't slept with someone for a long time.'

'I've always been careful when I've slept with

someone—and there are a lot fewer notches on my bedpost than rumour would have it,' Daniel said. 'Though it's your call.'

He was giving her the choice. Offering, not demanding. 'I'm happy to manage without,' she said.

He brushed his mouth briefly against hers. 'Then let me give you a guided tour of the house. You've already seen the living areas.'

And all of a sudden, she wasn't quite ready. She needed a little more time to strengthen her nerve. 'Though I've not browsed your book-shelves or looked at the photos on your mantel-piece,' she said.

As if understanding why she was suddenly backtracking, and wanting to reassure her that everything was fine and he wasn't going to pres-sure her, he said, 'Come through and look your fill.' He took her hand and led her through to the section with the sofas and the built-in book-shelves.

'Medical textbooks. Classic science fiction. Oh, and what's this?' She looked at the title of the book. '*Uncle Dan—This Is Your Life.*'

He smiled. 'The kids made it for me for my fiftieth birthday. With a bit of help from Mum, Ally and Colin, so they had access to the really embarrassing photos with me wearing terrible nineteen-seventies clothes.'

'May I?'

'Sure.'

She leafed through. There were photographs of Daniel as a baby and a toddler, and as a young child; his nieces and nephews had clearly had huge fun with the captions, mocking his fashion choices. Daniel as a scowling teenager with a terrible haircut. Daniel on the day he passed his driving test, the day he graduated and his first day as a junior doctor. Daniel clearly as the favourite uncle with his nieces and nephews, pushing them on the swings and helping them make sandcastles and chasing them with a garden hose in what she presumed was his parents' garden. Daniel with each of them on their graduation day, and what looked like their eighteenth and twenty-first birthdays as well, clearly taking them out for beer or cocktails. Daniel with smiling brides and grooms. And each page was filled with stories—filled with love.

The last page said it all.

May your half-century birthday be as golden as you are.
  We love you, Uncle Dan.
  Hannah, Milo, James and Daisy

'They obviously adore you,' Mandy said.

'It's absolutely mutual,' Daniel said.

There was a slight crack in his voice, and again she wondered if maybe he regretted not having children of his own. Not that she intended to hurt him by asking; if he wanted her to know, he'd tell her.

'That's lovely,' she said. She went over to the mantelpiece, which was crowded with photos of graduations and weddings. 'Clearly you're as close to your family as I am to mine.'

'Yes,' he said. 'I'm the baby, so obviously I was hugely annoying to Ally and Colin when I was little. But if I don't see them during any particular week we'll talk on the phone. We text each other all the time. And they know they can always stay here if they're coming up to London for an exhibition or a performance, or even just meeting friends and they want a bed for the night. Mum lives with Colin and Sasha by the sea in Sussex, and Ally and Jake live in a pretty village just outside Cambridge—Jake's just about ready to retire from teaching history.'

She noticed that Daniel didn't mention his dad. Had he, like her, been bereaved? Maybe he found it too hard to talk about. Now wasn't the time to ask.

'It's nice that you're close now,' she said.

'It is,' he said. 'Righty. Tour. We'll start at the top of the house—though I think we'll leave the roof terrace for today, because it's started lashing down with rain.'

'You've got a roof terrace?'

'It's a lovely place to sit on a summer evening. I've got a few pots of flowers up there, thanks mainly to Ally—she's the gardening guru of the family, and she's fixed me up with stuff I can more or less neglect and it'll still thrive,' he said. He ushered her up the two narrow flights of stairs to the top floor. 'This is the boxroom, really—it's where I keep my vinyl. I can't quite bear to get rid of it. But there's a sofa-bed there too, for guests.'

There was a cabinet with a turntable and amplifier on top; the shelves were filled with albums, and there were a couple of smaller boxes that looked as if they contained seven-inch singles. Another, much narrower, shelving unit contained CDs; and there were a couple of framed tour posters on the walls for bands from the nineties.

'Just remembering what I said downstairs,' he said, and quickly found the George Harrison's *Best Of* album. 'The first track. "Something". So it counts as George.'

'Raise you *Abbey Road*,' she said, with a grin. 'We could argue this until the cows come home.' She browsed through his albums. 'Oh, Dire Straits—I *loved* this album. I played mine to death.' She sang a snatch of 'Romeo and Juliet'. 'And you've got the older Fleetwood Mac stuff, not just the Lindsey and Stevie years. I approve.'

'Are you telling me we've got a similar music taste, too?' he asked.

'I think so. Led Zeppelin and Pink Floyd— Jen's three years older than me, and she got into them when her best friend's older brother played the classic tracks to her. And I wanted to do everything that Jen did, so I listened to them as well.'

'The more I get to know about you, Dr Cooke, the more I like you,' he said. He led her through to the other room, which held a wooden-framed bed and a matching pale wood chest of drawers; there were built-in storage cabinets, and a couple of beautiful watercolour landscapes. 'The guest bedroom,' he said.

On the next floor down was the bathroom, with a bath and separate shower; again, the room was beautifully light and very tidy.

He stood outside the last door. 'My room,' he said softly.

'Your space,' she said, equally softly. 'Your decision.'

For a moment, she thought he was going to lead her downstairs again, but then he opened the door.

The walls were painted the same pale sage

green as the rest of the house, again with water-colour landscapes on the walls. The floor was parquet, and there was a red Persian rug on the floor next to the bed. His sleigh bed was wide and looked incredibly comfortable, with deep pillows; there was a bedside cabinet next to the bed with a reading lamp, a book and a smart speaker. As with the other bedrooms, the storage was built in.

'Your house is lovely. And incredibly tidy, given how terrible you are about paperwork at the hospital.'

'I just hate paperwork,' he said. 'Everything here's tidy, because it makes my life easy. Though I do admit to having a cleaner. I want to spend my free time with my family and friends, not slogging through chores.'

'I'm not judging. My family and friends are important to me, too,' she said.

He took her hand and dropped a kiss into her palm, then folded her fingers over it. The sweetness of the gesture made her heart skip a beat.

'Whatever's going through your head right now, hold that thought,' he said quietly, and went over to the beside cabinet. A couple of moments later, the first notes of 'Romeo and Juliet' filtered into the room, making her smile. He switched on the bedside lamp, closed the Roman blind, then walked back over to her. Drawing her into his arms, he swayed with her to the first three lines of the verse, then crooned the fourth line into her ear.

It felt as if he meant it.

'Yes,' she said.

CHAPTER SEVEN

MANDY WOKE THE next morning, warm and comfortable, her head pillowed on Daniel's shoulder and her hand holding his against his chest.

'Good morning,' he said.

'Morning.' She pressed a kiss against his shoulder. 'What's the time?'

'Nearly nine,' he said.

'Then I,' she said, 'need to get home, shower and change. I'm due at my sister's for lunch.' Her hand tightened briefly round his. 'You're very welcome to join us, but I should warn you that my mum, my sister and my daughter will all grill you mercilessly.'

'I'm due at my sister's, too,' he said. 'Again, you're welcome to join us, but if you do I have a feeling there will be questions. Lots of them.'

'Let's both take a rain check,' she said, sitting up. 'And if you're off to Cambridge, you need to get going soon or you'll be late.'

'Can I get you some breakfast?' he asked.

'No, I'm fine,' she said. 'But thank you.' She

pulled on her clothes, and he found a pair of pyjama bottoms and pulled them on.

'I'll see you at work tomorrow, then,' he said, drawing her into a hug and kissing the top of her head.

'Yes.' She pressed her lips against his bare chest. 'Have a lovely day.'

'You, too.'

She was smiling all the way home. Daniel had been a generous lover; and instead of finding it shy and awkward, they'd laughed and enjoyed exploring each other. And afterwards they'd lain curled up in his bed, talking for hours, too comfortable to move. Eventually they'd pulled their clothes on and gone downstairs to eat leftovers from lunch for supper. And then he'd persuaded her to stay the night—not that she'd needed much persuading, because she'd enjoyed his company so much that she hadn't wanted to leave.

Thankfully she hadn't been needed at the hospital, and she'd finally gone to sleep in his arms.

It had definitely been worth breaking her rules.

Mandy was still smiling when she'd showered, changed and taken the other Greek walnut cake she'd made over to her sister's house.

'You look very happy today,' Jen remarked when she'd made coffee and they were sitting with their mother and Gemma in the living room; Dev was outside with Jen's husband Barry, looking at the classic car he was restoring. 'Is there something we need to know?'

Mandy wasn't ready to share her delicious secret, yet. 'No,' she said. 'I just had a good week at work.' She wrinkled her nose. 'Well, mainly. Monday was rough on all of us, and you don't need to know about that.' No way was she telling that particular horror story in front of her pregnant daughter. 'But Noah, the baby who came in with infant botulism last week, is responding well to treatment.' She smiled. 'Dan's including Noah's case in the next series, and there's a tiny interview with me because I'm the one who worked out what it was. And of course you both know better than to feed honey to a baby under the age of one, right?'

'Of course,' they echoed.

'So you're on very good terms with Dr Dan?' Jen raised her eyebrows.

'Everyone on the ward calls him Dan.' Mandy willed the blush to stay down. 'He's lovely to work with. So are the rest of the team. I'm glad I made the move to the London Victoria.'

Gemma gave her a searching look, and Mandy deftly switched the conversation to babies and when Gemma's next scan was due. Thankfully it seemed to distract her mum, her sister and her daughter, and she managed to keep the conversation on babies until lunch was ready.

'There's something different about you,' Ally said, narrowing her eyes and holding Dan at arm's length. 'You look…hmm…*relaxed*.'

'It's probably because we've just started filming. That always gives me an energy boost,' Daniel said.

'Hmm,' Ally said.

Daniel enveloped her in a hug. 'Plus I don't have to cook my own Sunday lunch today.' He gave her the roses he'd bought on the way to Cambridge, and a bottle of New Zealand Sauvignon Blanc.

'My favourites,' she said. 'Thank you.'

'My pleasure.' He handed over a packet of dog treats. 'Not forgetting Dora.'

The miniature dachshund, hearing her name, trotted over and nudged him with her nose. He bent down to scratch her behind the ears. 'Hello, gorgeous. You're nearly as gorgeous as my favourite sister.'

'Your only sister,' Ally said drily, but to his relief she let the conversation centre around her beloved dachshund.

He enjoyed the day, especially as his nephew and niece and their partners also turned up for lunch, and Ally suggested that as it was a lovely day they should all walk off the rice pudding with Dora in the grounds of the local stately home. The last bits of autumn colour sparkled in the late autumn sunlight, and the reflections in the river were stunning. This, he thought, was a place that Mandy would like.

He left his sister's house at the same time as the children, pleading Sunday night London traffic; back at the house, he texted Mandy.

Had a good day?

He debated putting a kiss, and decided that might be over the top, so he sent it as it was.

She texted him back within a minute.

Lovely. You?

Went for a walk after lunch.

He sent her the photograph of the woods reflected in the river, and one of Dora.

She rang him. 'That's gorgeous—and so's the dog.'

'Dora the Daxie. She's a sweetie,' he said.

'Where did you go?'

'A stately home near Ally's. Daisy and James were there, too, with their partners.' He paused. 'I had to use a few distraction techniques. Ally's first comment was that I looked *relaxed* and she wanted to know why.'

She chuckled. 'I had a similar problem.'

Oh, that chuckle. Right at that moment he really wanted to see her. But he didn't want to put pressure on her. 'Are you busy tomorrow night?'

'No—my book club's only on the first Monday of the month,' she said.

'Fancy joining me at the cinema? They're showing a season of nineties' films just round the corner from me. *Good Will Hunting* is on tomorrow evening.'

'I love that film,' she said. 'Yes, please.'

'I'll book tickets. It starts at eight, so we've got time to eat first,' he said.

'I'll look forward to it. See you tomorrow,' she said. 'Sweet dreams.'

'You, too,' he said.

At the hospital on Monday, they managed to act as if they were merely colleagues. Mandy was teaching, while Daniel was busy on the ward and in meetings. They left the hospital separately, took the Tube separately, met up at Sloane Street and walked to the French bistro Daniel had booked not far from the cinema.

The cassoulet and tarte tatin with Chantilly cream were both fabulous; but Mandy enjoyed Daniel's company even more. He was easy to be with, and she thoroughly enjoyed talking about favourite films and plays with him, particularly when she learned that his taste chimed with hers as much as their musical tastes did.

He held her hand through the film, and it made her feel as if she were a teenager, holding hands in the dark.

'Let me drive you home,' he said when they left the cinema. 'I know you're perfectly capable of getting the Tube, but I'm not quite ready to say goodnight to you yet.'

She felt the same way. 'All right,' she said.

They walked back to his street to collect his car, and he took the pretty route along Chelsea Embankment towards the Strand; the river reflected the lights from the bridges and the buildings and looked incredibly pretty. The narrow steeple of St Mary Le Strand rose up before them, brilliant white, followed by the iconic dome of St Paul's. Daniel didn't bother putting any music on through the car's sound system, because they didn't stop talking on the way, about anything and everything.

When they neared King's Cross, Mandy directed him to her address, and Daniel found a parking spot close to her flat.

'Would you like to come in for a coffee?' she asked.

'I'm incredibly tempted,' he said, 'but we both

have an early start tomorrow, so I'll say good-night now.'

This was their second date.

What now? Mandy wondered. Was his refusal to come in his way of preparing her for the last date? Would the next date be their last? Or would he, like her, break his rules and see where this thing between them went?

'Goodnight,' she said.

He kissed her lingeringly. 'I'll see you at work tomorrow. I know you have a class tomorrow night, but are you free on Wednesday evening?'

'Yes. You could come over and I'll cook for us,' she suggested.

'Thank you—I'd like that. I'll bring pudding,' he said. He took her hand, pressed a kiss into her palm and curled her fingers round it. 'See you tomorrow,' he said.

How did this man manage to make her knees turn to jelly, when nobody had done that since Laurence? she wondered. And it wasn't just that sweet little gesture of a kiss, but the fact that he waited until she'd let herself in safely through her front door before driving off. It made her feel cherished. She was perfectly capable of looking after herself, but it was nice to date someone who wanted to look out for her, too.

On Tuesday afternoon, Daniel caught up with her. 'Do you have time for a quick chat? I have a patient I'd like you to meet. He actually asked me if he could be on the show—he enjoyed telling me that his mum has a crush on me, and the poor woman turned beetroot—but, actually, I think he'd be a natural on television. He's also said that he's happy for the students to come and ask him questions, and I think he'd be an excellent case for them.'

'Sure,' she said. 'Can I have a patient history?'

'Joe Lavery, aged thirteen. If I tell you he's missing school because he's too exhausted to get out of bed, and he gets sharp pains in his stomach, what would you say?'

'I know what that makes me suspect, so I'd ask about bowel movements,' she said.

'There's diarrhoea and blood in his faeces,' Daniel said.

Which was what she'd expected him to say. 'Would I be right in guessing that he's very thin?'

Daniel nodded. 'His older brothers are tall and slim, but Joe's painfully slender, and his mum thinks he's stopped growing upwards. Joe himself says that he still has a baby face when some of his mates are starting to get fuzz, and he's not very happy about it because he thinks it'll put the girls off.'

'Bless him. Have you done an endoscopy and colonoscopy?' she asked.

'Yes. I've just had the results back. Want to see?' Daniel asked. At her nod, he brought up the images on his computer screen.

'Poor kid. He must've been in agony,' she said, seeing the extreme ulcerations from his throat right down to his anus. 'That's textbook Crohn's.'

'Which is why I thought of your students,' Daniel said. 'I'm going to admit him and put him on meal replacement drinks to help him gain weight. A couple of weeks of that, and then we can give him monthly infusions of infliximab to stop the inflammation.'

'Have you talked to him about the diagnosis?' she asked.

'He's round from the sedation now, so I'm just about to see him and his mum, if you'd like to join us.'

'All right. I'll just have a quick word with Kelly—' one of the other senior doctors on the ward '—and ask her if she'll keep an eye on the students for me, and I'll be with you.'

'I'll be in consulting room four,' Daniel said.

Once she'd made sure that her students all had someone to ask if they were stuck on anything— and told them they'd get to meet another patient shortly—she knocked on the door of consulting room four.

'Joe, Abigail, I'd like you to meet Mandy

Cooke, who job-shares with me,' Daniel said. 'Mandy, this is Joe Lavery and his mum, Abigail.'

Joe was very thin and pale, with a shock of blond curly hair and cornflower-blue eyes. Despite the fact that he was in obvious pain, he smiled at her. 'Hello.'

'Nice to meet you both,' Mandy said. 'Dan told me that you'd agreed to talk to my students. Thank you very much, Joe. I know it can be a bit embarrassing, so it's really appreciated.'

'It's important to talk about poo,' Joe said. 'Since I've been ill, my mates and I all talk about it more. You know, like if something doesn't feel quite right.'

'Talking's a good thing,' Daniel said.

'So did the camera tell you what's wrong with me?' Joe asked.

'Yes. We think you have Crohn's disease,' Daniel said. 'It's a sort of inflammatory bowel disease. Part of your gut becomes swollen, inflamed and ulcerated—that's why you get diarrhoea, blood in your poo and stomach pains, and why you feel tired.' He looked at Joe. 'Do you want to see the pictures?'

'Definitely,' Joe said.

Dan brought them up on the screen.

Joe's eyes widened. 'Wow. I wasn't expecting that.'

'You can definitely see why you're in pain,' Daniel said gently.

'What causes all the ulcerations?' Abigail asked. 'Is Joe allergic to any foods? And how do we know which ones?'

'Crohn's isn't caused by diet,' Mandy said. 'We don't know for sure what causes it. Sometimes it runs in the family.'

'Nobody else in our family has had any symptoms like Joe's, not even mildly,' Abigail said.

'Sometimes it's an autoimmune disease—that means your body's immune system, which defends you against infection, attacks your digestive system,' Daniel explained. 'Though, as Mandy said, we don't always know why it happens.'

'Can you cure it?' Joe asked.

'No. It's a lifelong condition, and it can be unpredictable,' Daniel said. 'You're likely to go into remission—that's when you feel really well—and at other times you'll have a flare-up, where your symptoms will be worse. The good news is that we can give you medicine to keep you in remission for long periods.'

'We can give you steroids, either as injections or a tablet, to calm the inflammation down,' Mandy said.

'Aren't they what body-builders use? The

dodgy ones, I mean, and they're angry all the time with Roid Rage?' Joe asked.

Mandy could see exactly why Daniel had suggested the teenager as a case study for her students as well as for his show. Joe was bright and slightly cheeky, even though he was obviously in pain, and she rather thought he'd enjoy testing the students. She smiled. 'It's a different sort of steroid. These are ones like your body produces naturally. Though they do have side effects— they can cause problems sleeping and make you more prone to picking up infection. You might find you put on weight.'

'That won't be a problem. I worry that he's all skin and bone as it is,' Abigail said.

'Sometimes steroids affect your growth,' Daniel said, 'so for the next couple of weeks we're going to put you on a liquid diet that contains all the nutrition you need. It'll help counteract that and help build your strength up.'

'Milkshakes?' Joe asked.

'Something like that,' Mandy said. 'We'll need to give you some biological medicines as well, when you've built up some strength.'

'Biological? Like laundry liquid?' Joe asked.

Mandy smiled. 'No. It just means they're medicines made from cell cultures rather than synthetically.'

'The one I want to prescribe is called infliximab,' Daniel said. 'The latest research shows that if we give it to you soon after diagnosis, you're less likely to need surgery in the future. We'll give you an infusion—that means we'll put you on a drip for a couple of hours so the medicine goes straight into your vein—and we'll need to do that once a month.'

'How does the medicine work?' Abigail asked.

'It's an antibody-based medicine and it targets a protein in your body called TNF-alpha—that stands for "tumour necrosis factor", but that isn't the same as cancer,' Mandy explained. 'TNF is naturally produced by your body and helps fight off infection, but too much of it can damage the cells lining the gut. What infliximab does is bind to the TNF-alpha and that reduces inflammation.'

'How long does it take to work?' Joe asked.

'Everyone responds differently. It might start helping straight away, or it might take two or three sessions,' Mandy said. 'We'll see how it goes, but if it suits you we'll suggest taking it for a year and then we'll review it.'

'Are there any side effects, like the ones with the steroids?' Abigail asked.

'There might be a bit of redness or swelling around the site where we give you the infusion, and you might get a headache or feel a bit sick,' Daniel said.

'You're also likely to pick up infections more easily,' Mandy added. 'We'll give you a leaflet so you know what to look out for, and you need to tell us if you've got a fever or you're worried about anything. I'd advise having a flu jab every year, and give us a call if you've been in contact with anyone who has chickenpox, shingles, measles or TB.'

'That's a big list of things,' Abigail said, looking daunted.

'I know it's a lot to take in. As Mandy said, we have patient information leaflets that can help you,' Daniel said, 'and we can also give you details of support groups. I know the diagnosis might feel like a bit of a shock right now, but there's no reason why Joe can't live a normal life. Yes, it's a lifelong condition and you'll need treatment, Joe, but that treatment will let you live a healthy life.'

'Thank you,' Joe said. 'So I can still play football, do computer stuff and see my mates.' He smiled. 'And, if I'm on telly, that means I might even get a girlfriend...'

CHAPTER EIGHT

ON WEDNESDAY EVENING, Daniel stopped at the deli round the corner from his house to buy a box of *macarons*, some out-of-season raspberries and a bottle of wine; he picked up a nice but not over-ostentatious bouquet of roses, gerbera and antirrhinum in autumn tones at the florist's, then caught the Tube from Sloane Square to King's Cross.

Mandy's flat was a short walk away, in a row of four-storey Georgian townhouses that were similar to his own but had clearly been split into flats. He pressed the button for her flat; a few moments later, he heard her voice. 'Hello?'

'It's Dan.'

'I'll buzz you in. Come straight up,' she said. Seconds later, he heard a buzz and a click, and he opened the front door.

Her flat was on the second floor, and she was waiting for him at the top of the stairs.

'Hi.' He kissed her cheek and handed her the bag with the wine, raspberries and *macarons*.

'For you. I'm afraid I cheated and bought pudding rather than making it.'

She looked inside the bag. 'Ooh, I love these. Thank you.'

'And also for you.' He gave her the flowers.

She smiled. 'They're beautiful. Thank you. Come through to the kitchen while I put the flowers in water. The bathroom's just here—' she indicated the door between what were clearly the living room and the kitchen '—if you need it.'

Her kitchen was square and compact, with pale primrose walls, beech cabinets, dark grey worktops and dark grey tiled flooring. There were a couple of pots of herbs on the windowsill, a wok set on the hob, and three bowls on the worktop next to it; one contained diced chicken, one contained diced vegetables, and one contained what looked like a home-made sauce. Next to them was a saucer containing grated fresh ginger and crushed garlic, and a wooden spatula.

He raised an eyebrow, smiling. 'You could be a TV cook, with everything prepped like that.'

She laughed. 'It just saves a bit of time. It'll take literally five minutes to cook this lot, boil the kettle and do some noodles to go with it.' She looked at him. 'Did you drive?'

'No. I came by Tube,' he said.

'Then there's a bottle of white wine already chilling in the fridge, if you'd like to pour us both a glass. Or I can offer you sparkling water, with or without elderflower; or make you some jasmine tea, if you'd prefer?'

'Jasmine tea?' He blinked.

She opened the door to the cabinet above the kettle. 'Behold my tea collection. Breakfast, Earl Grey, jasmine, peppermint, lemon and ginger, camomile and three different fruit teas.' She grinned. 'Gemma used to tease me about them.'

'Teasing about tea,' he said.

Her grin became a rich chuckle. 'Indeed. Anyway, when she fell pregnant and discovered she couldn't stand the smell of coffee, she was very grateful for my tea collection.'

'If you're having wine, so will I,' he said.

'The glasses are on the table in the living room,' she said, 'if you'd like to grab them.'

'Sure.'

Her living room was also square; there was a small table and four chairs placed against one wall, set with two places. A comfortable-looking dark red sofa sat opposite, with scatter cushions that matched the curtains of the two sash windows overlooking the street. Daniel recognised them as his sister's favourite William Morris design, in an elegant dark navy. The elegant fireplace was flanked on each side with shelves stuffed with a mix of what looked like medical textbooks and classic novels. He glanced at the photographs on the mantelpiece. One was clearly Mandy's daughter on her graduation day; one was Gemma's wedding; another was Mandy's own graduation day with her sister and her parents; and the final one was of Mandy as a bridesmaid. He guessed that the bride was probably Linda, her best friend.

Next to the sofa was a small table with lamp and smart speaker, and in the middle of the polished wooden floor was a navy rug with the same William Morris pattern as the cushions and curtains. Like the kitchen, the room was compact, but the overall effect was cosy rather than cluttered.

Mandy had put the flowers in a vase by the time he returned with the two wine glasses, and heated oil in the wok ready to cook the stir-fry.

He took the chilled bottle of wine from the fridge and poured two glasses of wine; he placed hers on the worktop next to the hob. He could smell the delicious aromas of the garlic and ginger sizzling.

'You have a very nice flat,' he said.

'Thank you. It's small, but it suits me—plus it has a spare bedroom next to mine, upstairs,' she added, 'which means I can have my grandchild to stay if Gemma and Dev are going out somewhere.'

She clearly had her life worked out, Daniel thought. He really wasn't sure if she would have room in her life for a relationship. Then again, neither did he. Besides, they'd both said that they didn't want a proper relationship. This was a fling, he reminded himself. For fun, not for ever.

He glanced at her fridge as he put the bottle back in to chill again. There were postcards stuck to the front with magnets, plus a couple of photographs, one of which appeared to be a group of people outside the Royal Opera House.

'Is that your ballet class?' he asked.

She glanced round to see what he was looking at, and smiled. 'Yes. We went to see *Swan Lake* together at Covent Garden earlier this year. We had amazing seats, and I think it was the best performance I've ever seen—everything was just perfect. We did the backstage tour, too, and it was fascinating. Did you know there used to be nine gin palaces on Bow Street? There's only one left now, though obviously it's a modern pub.' She grinned. 'And of course we had to visit it. We begged our teacher to do us a simplified bit of *Swan Lake* choreography, that half term.'

'What are the chances,' he asked, 'of you dancing it for me?'

'None, because I can't quite remember the

whole thing, now.' She smiled. 'But if you really want a demo, I can do you a simplified "Dance of the Sugar Plum Fairy". That's what we've been doing this term—obviously it's *Nutcracker* season.'

'I'm so in for that,' he said. 'Do you happen to have a tutu?'

She laughed. 'No. But I'll wear my practice skirt so you get the full effect of the swishy bits in the routine. After dinner.'

'I'll look forward to that,' he said.

As she'd suggested, it only took a few minutes to cook the stir-fry and the noodles. She served up, and took the bowls into the living room while he brought the glasses through.

'This is fabulous,' he said after the first mouthful.

'It's an easy recipe,' she said. 'From my favourite recipe website.'

As soon as she named it, he nodded. 'Mine, too. Which makes me sound horribly domesticated.'

'Nothing wrong with being capable,' she said.

He glanced up at the framed pictures of flowers on the wall. 'Is that cross stitch?' he asked.

'My guilty pleasure,' she said. 'I normally sew for an hour in the evening; it helps me decompress. I'm currently making a birth sampler for my grandchild.' She left the table to lift the cloth off a stand in the corner.

It was a charming design, with foliage in the shape of a heart and woodland animals peeping out of it—a fox, a squirrel, a rabbit and an owl—plus room in the centre of the heart for the baby's name and weight.

'Gemma and Dev chose a woodland theme for their nursery. I was so pleased when I found this pattern.'

'It's lovely,' he said. 'She'll be thrilled.'

'I hope so.'

He kept the conversation light, and insisted on helping her clear the table after they'd finished eating. Then he sneakily washed up while she went upstairs to change into her ballet clothes.

'You weren't supposed to do the washing up,' she said when she came back down to join him. 'I didn't wash up at your place.'

'You didn't need to. I have a dishwasher and a cleaner,' he reminded her.

'Even so. You're my guest. I should be waiting on you, not the other way round. Though thank you.' She rolled the rug up, to give her room to dance on the wooden floorboards. And she looked incredibly cute, he thought, in a black leotard, black footless dance tights, and a floaty chiffon skirt that reached down to just above her knees, plus pale pink ballet shoes.

'I need a two-minute warm-up so I don't pull a muscle,' she said, and proceeded to do what he assumed was the usual warm-up routine at her class. Then she switched on her smart speaker, connected it to her streaming service and called up 'Dance of the Sugar Plum Fairy'. The ethereal notes of the celesta shimmered in the air and she began to dance—not on pointes, as she'd already told him, but still on tiptoe. He was captivated by the graceful way she moved her arms and legs, the arabesques and turns, the tiny bourrée steps—and all with a smile on her face.

When the music ended, she swept into a deep curtsey, and he clapped.

'I loved that,' he said. 'You're amazing.'

She went pink. 'It's hardly in the same league as Sadler's Wells or the Royal Opera House. But I enjoy the music and the dancing. It's taken our class a while to learn this piece, even though it's only a couple of minutes long. And I'm sorry it's not the flashy one with all the fouettés and pirouettes that you've seen in a proper performance—this is a beginner's version.'

'I loved the routine,' he said again. 'And I love the way your skirt swished when you danced. It's given me all kind of ideas.'

'Oh, yes?'

He stood up and walked over to her. 'Do a twirl for me? Please?'

'I'm not very good at it, but I'll do you a soutenu turn,' she said. One leg came out, then as she drew her leg back in front of the other one she went on tiptoe, spread her arms, spun round and faced him with her arms posed above her head like a ballerina in a musical box.

'One more?' he begged.

She did so; this time, when she faced him again, he drew her into his arms and kissed her until she was breathless.

'Just as I dreamed it would be,' he said, his voice husky.

This time, she kissed him.

And he scooped her up and carried her up the stairs to her bedroom.

Afterwards, they lay curled in bed together.

'So tonight was pretty much our third date,' she said. 'Is this where you tell me that you've enjoyed my company but you'd rather we go back to being just friends—and I've done nothing wrong, it's just the way you are?'

Daniel gave her a wry smile. 'That's what I'd normally do, yes.' He paused. 'But you broke your rule for me by seeing me in the first place. I ought to break my rule for you.'

'But?'

The word that had echoed in his head; clearly

she'd noticed. 'You really are brave,' he said. 'Asking the difficult question.'

'It needs asking. And it does neither of us any favours if we sidestep it,' she said.

'All right. The thought of going past my three-date rule makes me antsy,' he said. Which was an understatement. It made his stomach turn to water. What if they kept seeing each other, got closer, and they fell in love? What if he let her down, the same way he'd let Roxy down? What if, deep down, he was still just like his father and he hadn't learned to be different?

The last thing he wanted to do was to hurt Mandy.

On the other hand, going back to being just colleagues and friends would be more than difficult, now. He really liked the woman he was getting to know. Liked her more than he'd liked anyone in a very long time. And she seemed to like him, too…

'Dan?' she asked gently. 'What do you want?'

To be sure I'm not my father's mini-me.

Not that he could explain that. Everything was too mixed up in his head. 'If I'm honest, the thought of not seeing you any more makes me antsy, too,' he admitted.

'So what do we do now?' she asked.

Panic? Oh, for pity's sake. 'I think maybe we

keep going until one of us is ready to say stop,' he said.

'And keep it just between us, for now,' she said.

'Just between us,' he agreed.

For the next couple of weeks, Mandy and Daniel sneaked in dates between work and her classes. Sometimes they went for a drink, sometimes they did the crossword together over a videocall, sometimes they went for a walk—and even on a rainy evening it was fun, holding hands and laughing as they dodged the puddles. He even let it slip to Ally that he was seeing Mandy. But on Saturday afternoon, when Mandy was sitting on Daniel's lap on her sofa and being thoroughly kissed, her phone rang.

She glanced at the screen. 'It's my daughter.'

'Answer it, or you'll worry yourself silly that there's a problem with the baby—and everything might be just fine,' Daniel said.

She nodded and answered the phone. 'Gemma? Is everything all right, darling?'

Gemma laughed. 'Don't panic, Mum. I've been shopping, and I found this incredibly cute cardigan for the baby, and I wanted to show you.'

Mandy closed her eyes in relief. 'That sounds great. Shall I come over tomorrow?' she asked.

'Actually, I went shopping not far from you and I'm nearly at your front door,' Gemma said.

'You're nearly at my front door now?' Mandy almost squeaked in horror.

That meant there wasn't enough time for Daniel to make a quick exit. But if Gemma saw him in her mother's flat, she'd ask questions. Questions that Mandy didn't know how to begin to answer.

Sorry, she mouthed at Daniel.

He mouthed back, *It's fine.*

'I'll put the kettle on. Is Dev with you?'

'No. It's just me,' Gemma said.

'All right. See you in a minute, sweetheart,' Mandy said, and disconnected the call. 'Sorry. I'll tell her you're just my friend. That you came over because you wanted to talk to me about something to do with the ward. Or about a case for your show—we could tell her about Joe.'

'Even though it's plausible, she's not going to believe a word,' Daniel said drily. 'Even if you comb your hair, you'll still look as if you've just been kissed until you're dizzy.'

She stared at him, and felt her eyes widen. 'That's how you look, too.'

He winced. 'Let's play this by ear. She might not notice.'

But of course she did. As soon as Gemma walked up the stairs and saw Daniel, and looked at her mother's face, she said, 'How nice to meet you, Dr Monroe. I enjoy watching your show. Mum, let me help you make that cup of tea.'

'It's not what you th—' Mandy began as Gemma bundled her into the kitchen and closed the door.

'No? You can't even meet each other's eyes,' Gemma said. 'You look like a pair of guilty teenagers.'

'How would you know?' Mandy retorted. 'You teach Reception class, not high school.'

'It's not that long since I was a guilty teenager myself,' Gemma reminded her. 'And it's pretty obvious you've just been snogging each other's faces off.'

Mandy groaned and rubbed a hand across her face. 'Oh, for pity's sake.'

Gemma hugged her. 'And I'm delighted you're seeing him. You know I worry about you being lonely. This will stop me fretting quite so much.'

'It's very, very early days,' Mandy warned. 'It might not come to anything. We're just seeing how things go.'

'If he makes you happy for now, that's enough for me,' Gemma said. 'Having said that, if he hurts you, he'll have me to deal with. In Mama Bear mode.'

Mandy hugged her daughter back. 'He's not going to hurt me, Gem. We're friends. Well, a little bit more than friends,' she admitted. 'Neither of us was expecting anything to happen, and we're finding our way round it.'

'Just live in the moment and enjoy it. It's about time,' Gemma said, and proceeded to take over making the tea, finding the biscuits and then shooing her mother out of the kitchen.

'Well?' Daniel whispered.

'We didn't get away with it,' Mandy whispered back. 'She says we look like guilty teenagers.'

He chuckled, and stole a kiss—just as Gemma brought the tea and biscuits through and caught them.

'The pair of you really have both regressed three and a half decades, haven't you?' she asked, but she was smiling.

'Born-again teenagers who are trying very hard to persuade everyone that they're just good friends but not making a very good job of it,' Daniel said cheerfully. 'Sorry, Gemma. Though I want you to know that I like your mother very much. She's a brilliant doctor and she's perfect as my job-share. I'm not going to do anything to jeopardise that. More importantly, even though neither of us really knows where this is going or what we want, I'm not going to do anything to hurt her.'

'Good,' Gemma said. 'Because you really

don't want an angry pregnant woman on your case, Dr Monroe.'

'Call me Dan,' Daniel said. 'And I hear what you say.' He paused. 'You're thirty-two weeks, aren't you?'

She nodded. 'I've been really lucky—I've only had a little bit of morning sickness.'

'That's good,' he said.

Gemma raised her eyebrows. 'I hear Mum's going to be on your show.'

'She's the one who spotted the infant botulism, so she deserves the credit,' Daniel said. 'Plus I like the way she teaches. Some of her students might end up on the show as well.'

Gemma chatted happily to both of them until she'd finished her tea. And then her eyes widened. 'I nearly forgot to show you the cardigan.' She rummaged in her shopping bag. 'Look. It's fleecy, and there are teddy bear ears on the hood.'

'That's seriously cute,' Mandy agreed.

'And I'd better get back before Dev starts worrying I'm late,' she said. 'It really was nice to meet you, Dan.'

'You, too,' he said.

'Have a good evening,' she said.

'Text me when you're home,' Mandy reminded her.

'I will. Don't fuss.'

Mandy laughed. 'Six months' time, it'll be me telling you not to fuss…'

'I'm a primary school teacher. Nothing fazes us or makes us fuss,' Gemma said, laughing back. 'But, yes, I'll text you when I'm home.'

'She's lovely. Very like you,' Daniel said when Gemma had gone.

'Thank you.' Mandy drew a breath. 'You do know she's going to be straight on the phone to her gran, her aunt and her godmother now she's left us, don't you?'

'Her godmother being your best friend?' he guessed.

She nodded. 'Gem will be telling them all about you. And there will be "casual" invitations.' She emphasised the word with finger quotation marks.

'So they can meet me and see for themselves if they're happy that I'll be good to you?' Daniel asked.

'Yes.' And the idea scared her witless. Until they knew where this thing between them was going, she'd rather keep it between themselves.

'I'm afraid my family will do the same kind of thing.' He paused. 'Maybe we ought to pre-empt it.'

She wasn't brave enough to do that. And she needed to be honest with him about it. 'I'm not sure I'm really ready for that,' she admitted.

'Me, neither.' Was that relief or trepidation she could see in his eyes? She wasn't sure. 'Perhaps it's better if we take each day as it comes and make excuses until we're ready.'

'That works for me,' she said.

The following week, on Tuesday evening, Mandy picked up a text from Daniel after her aerobics class.

Hope you had a good class. Ally's taking Jake to a show tomorrow night because the friend she was going with has flu. They want to have dinner with me—and you, too, if you're free. I can tell them I'm busy, or you can meet Ally and Jake. No pressure either way: your choice. D x

'Oh, help,' she said to Linda. 'What do I do?'

'What do you want to do?' Linda asked.

'Dan met Gemma at the weekend and they got on fine. Me meeting his sister would be the next step,' Mandy said. It meant taking their fling another step closer to being a proper relationship, and she wasn't entirely sure how she felt about that. Dan had swept her off her feet; she'd swept him off his feet, too. Were they ready for this, or had they already rushed everything and meeting each other's families properly would be a step too far? 'On the one hand, I'd like to meet her.' She bit her lip. 'On the other hand, what if she doesn't like me and thinks I'm completely wrong for Dan?'

Linda scoffed. 'The idea of anyone not getting on with you is so ridiculous, I'm not even going to dignify it with a response. Of course she'll like you.' She paused. 'I'd actually like to meet him, too. Obviously, only when you're ready.'

'I'm not sure I'm ready, yet.' Mandy bit her lip. 'This is ridiculous, Lin. I'm fifty-two years old and about to become a grannie. Yet I feel like a teenager, in a spin every time I think about him. I don't think I've ever blushed so much in my life, this last month or so.'

'You've been a brilliant mum to Gemma, a good support to your mum and your sister, and you're a legend among the students,' Linda said. 'You've put everything else on the back burner. Maybe it's time you put that part of your life first, just for a little while.'

'While my fling with Dan lasts, you mean?'

'Don't put limits on it,' Linda advised. 'Be open to…well, whatever happens. See where it takes you. You like him, and he likes you. Thinking about anything else will just overcomplicate it.'

'I guess…' Mandy texted him back.

Love to meet them. Let me know where and what time. M x

Half an hour later, her phone pinged with a message giving her the restaurant's address in Leicester Square.

Table booked for 6.15. (Their show starts 7.30) D x

On Wednesday, she and Daniel were both caught up in meetings all day and didn't get the chance to catch up with each other, but Mandy managed to get home in time to change into a little black dress before catching the Tube to Leicester Square. It was a short walk to the restaurant; when she gave Daniel's name at the reception, the waiter ushered her over to the table.

Daniel stood up, kissed her cheek, and seated her at the table. 'This is Ally, my sister, and Jake, my brother-in-law. Ally, Jake, this is Mandy.'

'Lovely to meet you,' Ally said.

'And you.' Daniel's sister looked like a feminine version of him, with the same deep brown eyes and dark hair shot through with grey, and she had the same warmth about her.

'How have you settled in at the hospital?'

'Really well. The team's great,' Mandy said.

'Dan said you were going to the theatre tonight.'

'It's a new production of *Oedipus*,' Ally said.

'I was going with a friend who teaches Classics at my school—I don't know if Dan told you I teach English at sixth form?—but she's gone down with a bug and I nagged Jake into coming with me because I didn't want to miss it. I asked Dan to meet us for dinner—and then it struck me, it'd be the perfect chance to meet you.'

'Thank you for asking me to join you,' Mandy said. 'Your dog's gorgeous, by the way. Dan showed me the photos he took from your walk.'

'Dora. Which is also short—like her legs—for "adorable",' Ally said with a grin.

'Excuse me. *I'm* the one who does the terrible jokes and puns,' Daniel interrupted.

'Believe me,' Jake said drily, 'your sister can give you a run for your money.'

'So can Mandy. Her daughter teaches Reception class,' Daniel said.

'Five's such a lovely age,' Ally said.

'Isn't it just? Though my source of jokes for my patients will be drying up for a little while,' Mandy said, 'when Gemma has the baby.'

'Is it her first?' Ally asked.

Mandy nodded. 'I'm so looking forward to being a grannie—in somewhere around seven weeks' time.'

'I would be, too,' Ally said. She smiled. 'It'll be a while until either of my two settle down and think about babies.'

'Daisy's the music therapy specialist and James is the archaeologist, right?' Mandy checked. 'Dan told me about them.'

'Thankfully they both live in London, so they're not that far from us,' Ally said. 'Dan's always been good with them. Especially Daisy—he got through to her when nobody else could.'

'I just did what you all would've done, if she'd let you,' Daniel said. 'She hated the pressure of her course. She would've made a good doctor, but she didn't enjoy it, and she simply needed someone to show her that she had options. That she didn't have to follow in anyone's footsteps and be a hospital doctor or a GP. She could still help people, but she could do it her way.'

'He took her to the beach for the day and made her walk for miles,' Jake said. 'And he told her to remember the little girl who used to dance and sing all the time. What did *she* want to do?'

'I wasn't trying to get her to drop out of uni and become a busker,' Daniel explained. 'But I said that there was a way she could use the music she loved in a medical setting. We talked about how some of my patients have play therapy, and how music therapy helps a whole range of people. I merely suggested that she could look into trying a different route that might make her happier.'

'Now she's working as a music therapist, and

she's got a research project about dementia and music,' Ally said proudly. 'But, most importantly, she's happy in her job. I hated seeing her trying to force herself into the wrong-shaped hole, and she was so stubborn about wanting to follow the family tradition of being a doctor. Her grandfather, her uncle and her cousin.'

Was it her imagination, Mandy wondered, or had Daniel flinched slightly when Ally mentioned their father? And he hadn't mentioned before that his dad had been a doctor. She wondered why. Had he not got on well with his dad?

'I wonder where Daisy gets her stubbornness,' Jake teased, nudging Ally.

She nudged him back. 'Some of it's from you,' she retorted.

They didn't have time for a pudding, and Daniel glanced at his watch and shooed his sister and brother-in-law from the table. 'My bill,' he said. 'Don't argue. You can treat me some other time. Go and enjoy the show.'

Ally hugged him warmly. 'Best baby brother ever,' she said. Mandy got a hug, too. 'The next weekend when you're free, come to Cambridge—with or without Dan—and we'll have that walk.'

'Definitely,' Mandy promised.

Then Ally murmured in her ear, 'I think you're good for him. Thank you for making him relax.'

That was incredibly cryptic, but there was no way she could ask for an explanation. At least, not when Ally and Jake had to get to the theatre in time to take their seats. Why would Daniel not be relaxed?

Clearly there was something else he hadn't told her. She didn't have a clue what it might be, or how to persuade him to open up to her. She'd just have to wait until he was ready.

She was still thoughtful after Ally and Jake had left, Daniel had paid and they'd gone back to her place for coffee because it had started to rain and her flat was nearer the Tube station than Daniel's was.

'You've gone quiet. Everything OK?' Daniel asked when they were curled up together on her sofa.

'It's fine,' she said with a smile. 'I liked your sister. She's very like you. Straightforward and easy to get on with. Jake seemed nice, too.'

'Yes, he is.' He dropped a kiss on the top of her head. 'I'm glad Ally didn't grill you. Mind you, she'd already asked me a lot of questions about you.'

'I think,' she said, 'our families think we're set in our ways and they worry about us.'

But were they too set in their ways, she wondered, for this thing between them to work? And what was Daniel holding back?

CHAPTER NINE

On Thursday, Mandy was working in the Paediatric Assessment section with one of her students when five-year-old Isabella Moran was brought in. The little girl was listless and had a temperature. Every so often, she coughed.

'She caught a cold at school,' her mum said, 'but she hasn't managed to shake it off. She's gone off her food, and last night her temperature spiked and I just couldn't get it down. And her breathing's funny, this morning. I rang the doctor and he told me to bring her straight here.'

'Absolutely right,' Mandy said. 'I'm Dr Mandy, and this is Tom, one of my students. Are you OK for Tom to sit in and maybe do some of the checks under my supervision?'

Isabella's mum nodded. 'I just want Bella to get better.'

'Let's have a look at you, sweetheart,' Mandy said, lifting the little girl onto the examination couch. Her temperature was just over thirty-nine centigrade, and her breathing was faster than

Mandy was happy with. 'Is it all right if Tom and I have a listen to your breathing with our stethoscopes? When we're done, you can listen to Mummy, if you like.'

The little girl didn't even smile or nod, just looked weary, and the anxiety in her mum's face grew deeper.

'It might feel a little bit cold on your back,' Mandy warned.

Isabella's mum lifted the little girl's sweater at the back so Mandy could listen.

'Can you do me a big breath in and a big breath out, please, Isabella?' Mandy asked.

The little girl did so. As Mandy had suspected, she could hear crackles: a bubbly sound, like Velcro being ripped open. But, more worryingly, she could hear a pleural rub as well.

'Tom?'

Her student placed his stethoscope in the same place that Mandy had. 'Big breath in for me, please, Isabella?' he asked. 'And out?' He frowned and looked at Mandy. 'It sounds bubbly,' he said. 'That's coarse crackles, right?'

She nodded. 'And what causes that?'

'Mucus in the bronchi—that's the tubes that connect your windpipe to your lungs,' he said.

'Did you hear anything else?'

He frowned. 'Not sure.'

'Something a bit like a snore crossed with someone walking in fresh snow?' she suggested.

Tom listened again. 'Yes, but I don't know what that is.'

'It's called a pleural rub, or sometimes a friction rub,' Mandy said. 'Mrs Moran, given that Isabella's temperature's still high, her breathing's fast and she's coughing, I think she has pneumonia. We can treat that, but I want to send her for a chest X-ray and possibly an ultrasound as well, because I think she has an infection.'

'Will she have to stay in, or can I take her home again?' Mrs Moran asked.

'That depends on the X-ray,' Mandy said. 'I'll be able to give you a better idea after that's done.'

She sent Tom with Isabella for the X-ray, then reviewed the images with him and sent him off to sort out an ultrasound. When the results were back, she went to see Isabella and her mum.

'She's got a condition called empyema,' Mandy said. 'Normally, the narrow space between your chest wall and your lungs is filled with pleural fluid. When you have pneumonia, the amount of fluid increases faster than it can be absorbed, and it gets infected.' Usually with *Streptococcus pneumonaie* or Group A Strep; she thought of baby Aarya and sighed inwardly, though she was careful not to let any of her sadness show. 'The infection causes the fluid to form pockets of pus, which coat the outer layer of the lungs and stop them expanding properly so it's harder for someone to breathe. The X-ray shows those little pockets of pus on Isabella's lungs, so we need to treat that. With young children, we tend to try conservative management first. I'm going to get her to cough up some sputum and I'll get the sample tested to find out which bacteria's involved, but it does take a couple of days to grow the culture, so in the meantime I'll give her broad-spectrum antibiotics on a drip. She'll be able to walk about and do things—we encourage that—as long as you're careful not to let her knock the drip. We'll keep her in for a couple of days and see how she responds to them; if she seems a bit better, you can take her home to finish the antibiotics in tablet form.'

'What if she doesn't get better?' Mrs Moran asked.

'Then we'll need to insert a tube called a chest drain to get the fluid and pus out,' Mandy said. 'It's something the paediatric surgeon will do under a general anaesthetic or sedation, so she won't feel any pain. Then she'll stay in for another three or four days, until the infection has cleared and her lungs are fully expanded again, and her temperature's down. But we'll start the antibiotics now, and Tom will take you both to the ward to settle her in. I'll pop in after clinic to see how she's doing, but if you're worried about anything have a word with one of the nurses. They're all really lovely and good with little ones. And if they're worried about anything they'll come and get me.'

The following day, during ward rounds, Mandy noted that Isabella hadn't shown any signs of improving.

Mrs Moran was at her daughter's bedside. 'Is Bella getting better?' she asked.

'Not according to her charts.' Mandy gave her a sympathetic smile. 'We'll need to get the surgeons to put a chest drain in.'

'You told me about that yesterday.' Mrs Moran looked anxious. 'An operation.'

'They'll use a really light anaesthetic so she'll come round very quickly,' Mandy reassured her. 'Once it's in, we'll put a dressing on to keep the area clean. It's sometimes a little bit uncomfortable so we'll make sure she has pain relief. And as the pus drains out she'll find it easier to breathe.' She paused. She'd mentioned Isabella to Daniel, yesterday, and he'd said that it sounded like a potential case for the show and asked if she'd mind introducing him. 'My colleague Daniel Monroe presents the *London Victoria Children's Ward* series. Would you consider having a chat with him about maybe including Isabella's case in his show?'

'She'd be on television?' Mrs Moran's eyes widened.

'It'd be just a chat at this stage,' Mandy said. 'But he's very keen on including the kind of cases we see quite often, as well as the rare ones. Seeing Isabella would help other parents to keep an eye out for the symptoms of pneumonia and maybe get treatment earlier than they would've done—as well as reassuring them that lots of other children go through this and get better.' She smiled. 'Dan's really nice. Apart from being a good doctor, he really cares, and children respond to him. I've seen him read stories to comfort a tearful toddler, and tell terrible jokes to make a teenager laugh.'

'I watch the show,' Mrs Moran said. 'He comes across as really lovely.'

'He is,' Mandy said, and meant it. Daniel was the kind of man who made the world feel like a better place.

Mrs Moran nodded. 'All right. I'm happy to have a chat with him.'

'Thanks. I'll go and have a quick word with him when I've finished ward rounds, and I'll introduce you to him,' Mandy said.

* * *

'Pneumonia and empyema,' Daniel said when Mandy had finished giving him a quick rundown. 'And we're looking at a chest drain, so with the parents' permission we can film in Theatre,' he added thoughtfully. 'Parents get twitchy about anaesthetic and sedation. It'd be nice to be able to reassure them and show them what happens.'

'I've spoken to the surgical team and they're going to put the chest drain in this afternoon,' Mandy said. 'And Mrs Moran says she's happy to have a chat with you. Is now a good time to introduce you?'

'Yes,' Daniel said. Shalmi, Carey and Keisha were busy examining the footage they'd already taken that morning and making notes about what they needed to film to complete the story. 'OK for me to dip out for a few minutes to talk to the mum of a potential case?' he checked with Keisha.

'Fine,' she said with a smile.

'Great. See you soon.'

Daniel walked with Mandy to Isabella's bedside, where she introduced him to Mrs Moran and Isabella.

'Hello, Isabella. I'm Dr Dan,' he said, sitting on the edge of her bed. 'I work with Dr Mandy. She tells me you're feeling poorly.'

The little girl nodded.

'We're going to make you feel much better,' he promised. 'I see your mum has been reading you one of my favourite stories ever. I used to read this book to my nieces.' He gestured to the book about a ballet-dancing mouse. 'Can I read a bit to you?'

The little girl looked to her mum, who smiled. 'If you'd like that, Bella, it's fine.'

'You like ballet?' Dan asked.

Isabella nodded.

'She goes to lessons,' Mrs Moran said. 'She's missing it at the moment.'

'My niece Daisy did ballet lessons, too, when she was your age,' Dan said. 'And she still remembers me reading this story to her.' He read a little bit of the book, doing a special squeaky voice for the mouse when she talked, and Isabella smiled.

He finished the page, and gave the book back to her. 'I'll read you a little bit more later, if you like.'

The little girl looked pleased. 'Thank you.'

'And I'll tell you a secret, Bella,' Dan said in a stage whisper. 'I know someone else who does ballet. Someone standing right near us. Can you guess who?'

'Mummy?'

'Your mummy dances, too? That makes *two* other people, then.' He added in a stage whisper,

'Dr Mandy goes to ballet lessons.' Then he gave an exaggerated frown. 'Oh, dear. That means I'm the only person here who doesn't do ballet. You know what? When you're feeling better, maybe you can teach me how to do a ballerina twirl.'

Isabella gave a tiny giggle, and he laughed back. 'Bella the Ballerina, and Dan the Dancer. We're going to be a great team. Give me a high five.'

The little girl did so.

'Now, I'm going to have a chat with Mummy.' He glanced at Mandy.

'And I'm going to take over reading, though I'm not as good at the voices as Dr Dan,' Mandy said. 'Can you show me which is your favourite picture, Isabella?'

Daniel ushered Mrs Moran a few metres away, so Isabella wouldn't overhear but was still in her mother's view.

'That's the first time I've heard her giggle in a week,' Mrs Moran said. 'Thank you. That's amazing.'

'I remember having my tonsils out when I was only a year or two older than Bella,' he said. 'I didn't feel very well, and I didn't know how to explain how I felt. And hospital was *horrible*. Everyone had to be really quiet, there were weird smells and beeps that I didn't understand, and nobody smiled. When I became a doctor, I was determined that my ward wouldn't make children feel worse, the way I'd felt when I was small.' He smiled. 'That's why I have a stock of terrible jokes and a book of stickers in my pocket. I know a couple of basic magic tricks, too. But when children have favourite books, that makes it easier for me to connect with them and reassure them.'

'Dr Mandy said you might want to include Bella on your show.'

'With your permission, obviously. And we'd have a chat with you as well, to get the parent's point of view.'

'I'm not sure I'd be any good on television,' Mrs Moran said.

'My production team are brilliant,' Dan said. 'It's not all the scary, glamorous stuff. We film ordinary people who know what it feels like to worry about their child. The show's about reassuring other parents that how they're feeling is normal, and other families have been through it and come out the other side. And you don't have to learn a script or read cue cards—it'll be like sitting on a sofa in your living room, having a cup of tea and a chat with me. Just like we're chatting now.'

'You made my Bella smile,' Mrs Moran said. 'So all right, we'll do it.'

'Thank you,' Daniel said.

* * *

Later that afternoon, Isabella had been to Theatre; the chest drain was in place, along with urokinase, a clot-busting drug that helped to break up the pus. The little girl was asleep when Mandy checked in on her but appeared to be breathing a little more easily, to Mandy's relief.

Mrs Moran couldn't stop talking about how wonderful Daniel was. 'You were right. He's lovely,' she said. 'You've been lovely, too, but there's something so calming about him. And the way he read to Bella and chatted to her about ballet and made her brighter than she's been in a week—I bet he's a wonderful dad.'

Except Daniel didn't have children, Mandy thought. Because he'd never let anyone close enough to him to make a family, after his divorce. 'All the children on the ward love him, from the toddlers to the teens,' she said instead. 'He makes time for them, and that's important.' She smiled. 'Did you enjoy the filming?'

'Surprisingly, yes. Dr Dan was right; it really was like having a cup of tea and a chat in my living room.'

'If I know Dan,' Mandy said, 'there was tea or coffee involved. And biscuits.'

'Chocolate ones,' Mrs Moran confided.

Mandy smiled. 'Excellent. I'll pop in and see

how she's getting on tomorrow. The sputum test probably won't be back, but I'll check anyway.'

'It's your weekend on shift?' Mrs Moran asked.

'No. The nice thing about being a senior consultant is that I'm on call alternate weekends, but I don't have to come in unless I want to say hello to a special patient,' Mandy said with a smile. 'And Bella counts as special.'

Daniel met Mandy at her flat after ballet class.

'Sorry if I put you on the spot with Isabella, earlier, when I told her about your ballet lessons,' he said.

She smiled. '"Spot" has a very different meaning in a dance class; you look at a spot on the wall when you do a turn and make sure you keep looking at the same place. It helps you control the movement, keep your balance and prevent dizziness.'

'Am I going to get a demo?'

'From Bella, maybe,' she teased. 'Dan the Dancer.' She couldn't help a chuckle. 'Perhaps I should teach you how to do a pirouette, or at least a kind of turn.'

'If I can let Daisy and Hannah put sparkly slides in my hair and paint my nails, then I can learn to do a pirouette for a poorly little girl.'

He'd been that patient with his nieces? Then

again, she wasn't surprised. She'd discovered that Dan had a very soft centre, behind the charm and the humour. 'All right,' she said. 'I'll teach you.'

'Wearing that swishy skirt?' he asked, sounding hopeful. 'It'll help me concentrate.'

'Oh, really?' she teased.

He grinned. 'Busted. I just like seeing you in your ballet clothes. And I like thinking about how I can unwrap you, afterwards.'

'You have to earn that,' she warned.

'Change back into your ballet stuff,' he said, 'and teach me.'

'Roll the rug back while I change,' she said. 'And you need to be in socks. Roll them down over your heel to the middle of your arch, so you can slide on your toes and use your heels to stop yourself sliding.'

He gave a little hum of pleasure when she was ready. 'Have I told you how hot you look in that skirt, Dr Cooke?'

She laughed. 'I think I've got the message. Right. We're going to warm your muscles up first. I assume you've gone to some kind of exercise class in the past and know you just mirror the teacher?'

'Yes,' he said.

She got him to roll his shoulders forward and back, singly and together, and then taught him the basic arm movements of ballet. 'Make it flow,' she said. 'And now I want your arms up, in fifth position. Just how children do when you're playing "Simon Says" and tell them to put their arms like a ballerina's.'

He did so. 'Is that right?'

'Pretty much. I'm not going to fuss about your fingers.'

'What's wrong with my fingers?' he asked.

'I'll let Bella tell you,' she said. 'And now I want you on your tiptoes. Right foot in front of your left, feet close together. Keep looking straight ahead, and you're just going to take tiny steps—that's a bourrée,' she said. 'Turn as you step. Tiny, tiny, tiny steps.'

'That wasn't a pirouette,' he said, when he'd turned round and she'd said he could stand on flat feet again.

'It's nearly as good as one,' she said. 'It'll be good enough for Bella to enjoy it.' She gave him a wicked grin. 'And I might just mention it to Keisha.'

'I'll do this for Bella, but *not* for the show,' he warned.

She spread her hands. 'If you can let a child put sparkly clips in your hair... Hey, if you do a pirouette, they might even ask you to go on *Strictly*.'

'No. I only do celeb stuff if it's going to benefit the hospital. And now I claim my reward,' he said. 'Unwrapping you.' He pulled her to him, undid the bow she'd tied to keep her dance skirt in place, and slowly spun her round as he unwrapped her skirt. 'You're doing bourrées,' he said, narrowing his eyes at her.

In answer, she put her arms up, the way she'd just taught him to do, and hummed a bit of the Sugar Plum Fairy.

His retort was to scoop her over his shoulder in a fireman's lift and carry her up the stairs to her bed.

Afterwards, he went down to raid her cupboards and fridge for cheese and crackers, and brought a glass of wine with the plate to share.

'Are you staying tonight?' she asked.

'If you're asking.'

She kissed him lightly. 'I'm asking.'

'Then I'm staying,' he said softly.

CHAPTER TEN

THE NEXT MORNING, Daniel woke before Mandy. Her head was pillowed on his shoulder and her arm was wrapped tightly round his waist. And this felt oh, so right.

He'd been seeing her for a month now, and it felt as if he'd known her for always.

In some ways, it worried him. This was getting way too close to a proper relationship—something he'd avoided for years. He'd never forgive himself if he hurt her. Maybe he should back off. Take things a little more slowly. Be really, *really* sure about what he was doing.

On the other hand, waking with her in his arms made the mornings feel brighter. It was the perfect start to the day. Maybe he should brush his worries aside. After all, he was older now, and much wiser than he'd been when he'd wrecked his marriage. And what if Mandy was the person he'd been waiting to share his life with?

He wanted to believe in love. Yet at the same

time it scared him stupid that this relationship was going to go wrong. That he'd let her down, the way he'd let Roxy down. That deep down he was just as bad as his father had been and he'd never be able to settle.

Eventually she stirred. 'Good morning.'

And there it was, the almost shy smile that took his breath away and made him forget his worries. 'Good morning,' he said. 'What do you want to do today?'

'I'm on call,' she said.

'If it's a major emergency,' he reminded her. 'There are other consultants who'd be called in before you.'

'True. But I want to pop in to the ward, this morning.'

'To see how Isabella's doing?' he guessed.

'And to check on the sputum culture results. They probably won't be there until Sunday, but it's worth a look, just in case,' she said.

He stroked her hair from her face. 'You know, if it is Group A strep, rather than *strep pneumoniae*, we're not going to have a repeat of what happened to Aarya. Bella's a lot older and her system's strong enough to cope.'

'I know,' she said lightly.

'But you worry anyway,' he said. And that was what made her a good doctor. Attention to detail. Making sure things were checked. 'Do you want me to come in with you?'

'No,' she said. 'Because then people might put two and two together.'

He knew she was being sensible. They weren't going public with what was happening between them; only their closest family and friends knew. But at the same time it made him feel like a dirty little secret; and again his doubts flooded back. Was this all a huge mistake? Was he kidding himself that he could make it work? Was he expecting too much of himself? 'I'll go home and shower and change,' he said. 'What do you want to do after you've seen Bella?'

'What's the weather forecast?' she asked. 'If it's wet, then something indoors. If it's dry, it'd be nice to go for a walk.'

He checked the weather forecast app on his phone. 'Dry. How about Hampstead?'

'The Heath?'

'Sort of,' he said. 'It's an unusual garden. And then maybe we can have lunch in Hampstead and wander round the shops.' Somewhere public. Somewhere with no pressure. And maybe he could stop himself worrying that it was all going to go wrong. Stop himself worrying that he couldn't be the man she needed him to be.

'Sounds perfect,' she said.

* * *

After breakfast, Mandy went to the hospital while Daniel went back to Chelsea; they agreed to meet on the platform for the Jubilee Line at Westminster.

At the London Victoria, Mandy discovered that the sputum culture results weren't back yet, but Isabella had a little more colour in her cheeks and wasn't coughing quite so much. Plus, to Mandy's relief, Isabella's breathing seemed to be easier. 'It looks as if she's turning the corner,' she said to Mrs Moran.

'I hope so,' Mrs Moran said feelingly.

'You look exhausted,' Mandy said gently. 'I know you want to be with her, but I promise the team here will look after her tonight. Go home and get some proper rest.'

Mrs Moran sighed. 'I know that'd be the sensible thing to do—but she's my only one, and I can't bear to leave her.'

'I get that,' Mandy said. 'My daughter's my only one, too.' She squeezed Mrs Moran's hand. 'But, seriously, the best way to help look after her is to look after yourself. Go home and get some sleep. We'll ring you straight away if she wakes and calls for you, or if we're worried that her condition's worsening—though that's unlikely, now, as she's responding to the treatment.'

'Maybe I will,' Mrs Moran said.

'It's your choice,' Mandy said. 'But my advice—as a doctor and as a mum—is to get some proper rest tonight.'

Daniel was waiting for Mandy at Westminster station.

'How's Bella?' he asked.

'Her breathing's better, the cough's improving and she's got more colour in her cheeks. Though the sputum culture results aren't back yet.'

'She's got another day and a half of urokinase,' he said, 'and we'll know on Monday if we need to change to a more narrow-spectrum antibiotic. I think we can safely say she's on the way to recovering.'

'Agreed,' she said.

They got off the Tube at West Hampstead, then walked through Golders Hill Park, hand in hand, enjoying the last of the autumn colours. It had rained overnight, so the trunks of the trees were very dark and the brightness of the sun made the yellow leaves stand out.

'"That time of year thou mayst in me behold,"' Daniel quoted.

She smiled and chimed in with him. '"Where yellow leaves, or none, or few, do hang."'

OK, so the Shakespearean sonnet was one of the most famous ones: but even so they seemed to be finishing each other's sentences, she thought. Their minds seemed to work the same way. She'd never felt like that with anyone before, even Laurence; maybe, just maybe, her family and friends had a point after all and she'd been missing out by cutting relationships out of her life.

Or maybe, a little voice said in her head, maybe she'd just been waiting for the right person to walk into her life. Even though, technically, she'd walked into his.

They wandered past the small zoo and the playground. 'I'm looking forward to enjoying the toddler years again with my grandchild,' she said. 'The swings and the slides, and a little face all bright with excitement.'

'I think the beach is still my favourite place to take kids,' he said. 'Building sandcastles with a moat, splashing in the sea, and peering in rockpools. And I'll never forget the time we had a family holiday up in Yorkshire with all of us staying in this huge converted barn. James must've been about seven at the time. He'd always been into dinosaurs, and he begged us to take him fossil-hunting. We went to the beach at Staithes, and he rushed ahead, desperate to be the first one to find an ammonite.' He laughed. 'He was indeed the first to find an ammonite—but what we all remember more is that he jumped up and down in utter joy with his hands held up in triumph...and then he slipped and landed bottom-first in a puddle! He's never quite lived it down.'

Again, Mandy thought what a good father Daniel would've made. She knew he was wary of relationships after the break-up of his marriage, but he'd denied himself something so special. Why hadn't he believed in himself?

'I can just imagine it,' she said. 'We never managed to find any fossils when Gemma was small, but we used to go to the Natural History Museum on a very regular basis to see the dinosaurs.'

'That was James's favourite place, too,' he said. 'And I can remember building a balsa wood *Tyrannosaurus rex* with him.'

'Oh, look—fallow deer,' she said, pointing over to the trees, where a small group of fallow deer were grazing, their deep russet coat dappled with pale spots. 'They're gorgeous. The park here is definitely going on my list of places to bring the baby.'

A narrow path had them crunching over the fallen leaves of orange and russet and gold; at the end there were metal railings leading to a wrought iron gateway, and there were elegant stone columns topped with wooden trellises. Ivy twined round the columns, and climbing plants that she didn't recognise, full of richly coloured berries.

'That's gorgeous. I didn't expect it to be like this,' she said.

'It was built by Lord Leverhulme at the beginning of the last century as a place to entertain his guests and hold summer parties,' Daniel told her. 'Did you know, the pergola itself is as long as Canary Wharf tower is tall?'

'Been reading a guidebook, have we?' she teased.

'Websites,' he admitted. 'I wanted to know a bit more about the place. Guess what it's built on?'

She could see his eyes glittering with amusement, and remembered what they'd been talking about earlier. 'Dinosaurs?'

'Nope,' he said. 'It's the debris from where they dug out the extension of the Northern Line to Hampstead. The designer used the rubble to raise the hill and make the terraces.'

They climbed up the steps to the pergola and wandered through the walkways; there was a stunning view of the red brick arches supporting the pergola, and the formal terraced gardens below.

'Apparently it's really pretty in spring, with loads of wisteria,' Daniel said, 'and in the summer it's full of roses.'

'I can just imagine Edwardian garden parties here, the women all in elegant dresses and sipping champagne from coupe glasses,' she said. 'A string quartet playing…' She smiled. 'I loved all the Merchant Ivory films from the eighties.'

'This place was all pretty much in ruins, back then,' he said, 'or it would've made a good film set.'

Once they'd had their fill of the gardens, they headed down through the heath to Hampstead itself.

The village was seriously pretty with narrow winding streets; there were Regency townhouses with sash windows and gorgeous metal porches with trellised stands supporting roses and climbing shrubs; the shopfronts were picture-postcard, each one different, and a mixture of everything from florists to upmarket grocers to antique shops.

'All that walking's made me hungry,' Daniel said.

They found a little café, and ate a fabulous roasted tomato and red pepper soup served with artisanal bread and excellent coffee. Once restored, they continued wandering through the little side streets. They spent a while browsing in a second-hand bookshop; Mandy found a collection of Daphne du Maurier short stories she hadn't yet read, while Daniel came out with a volume of Cornell Woolrich's short stories.

'I've not read anything by him,' she said.

'He was one of the pulp fiction authors of the nineteen-forties,' Daniel said. 'A few of his stories were made into films—you'd definitely know *Rear Window*.'

'The Hitchcock film?' At his nod, she smiled. 'I love the James Stewart films.'

'Including the best Christmas film ever,' he said.

'I watch *It's a Wonderful Life* every year,' Mandy confessed. 'It always makes me a bit sad and cross at the very end, though, because Henry Potter gets away with stealing the money.'

'But money and greed can't buy him the love that the people of Bedford Falls give George Bailey for being the man at the heart of their community. George stood up to the bully and he prevailed. Potter has to live with knowing that,' Daniel pointed out. 'And his plans for Pottersville never happen.'

'I would just have liked a bit more justice. And for Potter to apologise to George,' Mandy said.

'But it wouldn't have been a genuine apology. It would've been lip service,' Daniel said. 'How do you even start to apologise when you've done that much wrong to someone?'

There were shadows in his eyes that made

Mandy wonder if he was talking about himself. But surely he'd paid his debt to Roxy, with that life of loneliness—never letting anyone close? She tightened her fingers round his. 'I think if you're genuinely sorry, it shows. And it changes you for the future. You learn from your mistakes,' she said.

'Maybe.' He didn't sound as if she'd convinced him, but he distracted her from taking the conversation further by pointing out an old-fashioned toy shop. 'Detour alert. I have something I need to buy.'

She raised an eyebrow. 'For your nieces and nephews?'

'No. For the kids on the show. I normally buy them a little something, just a token, to say thanks for their help.' He smiled. 'I'm still in touch with the kids from the first series. Even the ones who aren't still treated by our department, because their parents send me a Christmas card to the hospital every year with a photo and an update.'

'That's lovely,' she said.

Looking round the shop, Mandy found the softest, cutest little white rabbit and couldn't resist buying it for her grandchild-to-be. And Daniel was delighted to find a mouse dressed in ballet shoes and a tutu. 'This is perfect for Isabella,' he said.

'And you know what you have to do when you give it to her. Even if you do it in your normal shoes,' she said.

In response, he stood on tiptoe with his arms up, and did the turn she'd taught him, not caring that they were in the middle of the shop and people were staring.

'Perfect,' she said, clapping her hands.

Mandy was beginning to think that maybe this time she'd got it right, because Daniel was one of the good guys. A man with a huge heart who cared about his family, who supported his colleagues, and who tried to make a difference to people's lives with his television work as well as his hospital work.

Could she trust him with her heart?

Yes, he'd made a huge mistake, all those years ago. He hadn't fought hard enough to save his marriage to Roxy, and he'd let himself be dazzled by Leila. He'd broken the vows he'd made before his family and friends, to love and honour and cherish—just as Laurence had broken his vows to Mandy.

But Daniel wasn't like Laurence. He truly regretted what he'd done: to the point where he'd never put himself in a position where he could hurt someone again.

Though it had all happened half a lifetime ago. He wasn't the same man now who'd married Roxy and cheated with Leila. So maybe it was safe to take the risk that he wouldn't cheat on her. Safe to ask him to make a proper go of things.

'What do you want to do this evening?' she asked. 'Do you want to eat out, or shall I cook for us?'

'It's my turn to cook,' he said. 'Let's pick up something while we're here.'

And of course they ended up in the bakery section of the deli. 'Blueberry polenta cake,' Daniel said, looking gleeful. 'Does that work for you?'

'That'd be lovely,' she said. 'Though pudding and wine will be my contribution to dinner.'

Back at Daniel's house, Mandy enjoyed sitting at the table chatting to him about books while he cooked, sipping a glass of perfectly chilled Sauvignon Blanc, with gentle classical music playing in the background.

Dinner was perfect: chicken in a tarragon and crème fraiche sauce, served with roasted Mediterranean vegetables and fluffy basmati rice, followed by the polenta cake and vanilla ice cream.

And then they curled up on the sofa together.

'Shall we watch *It's a Wonderful Life*?' he suggested.

'Great idea.' She smiled. 'Especially as you've

taught me to look a little bit differently at the ending—at the bit that bothers me.'

'I'm glad,' he said.

She stole a kiss. 'You've taught me to look at other things differently, too.'

'How do you mean?' he asked.

This was a risk. But it was one she was willing to take. 'About dating someone. This last month, I've had such a good time with you.' She took a deep breath. 'I like who you are, Dan, and I think you like me, too.'

Ice slithered down Daniel's spine. He had a nasty feeling he knew where this was going.

Her next words confirmed it.

'I want to change the terms of our fling,' she said. 'I'd like this to be a real relationship. And I was thinking, I know you've already met Gemma, but maybe tomorrow you'd like to come for lunch and meet my family properly.'

A real relationship.

Meet her family properly.

The words screeched like an alarm in the back of his head.

This would mean a relationship without strictly defined boundaries—and he brushed aside the fact that that was exactly what had been happening since their first week together. There was a huge difference between saying they were seeing where something was going, keeping things on a more or less casual basis, and officially dating where everyone knew about it.

What if things went wrong?

It was incredibly brave of Mandy to suggest taking such a risk on a proven cheat, when her marriage had broken up because of her ex's infidelity. Daniel knew he wouldn't be carelessly unfaithful to her. But he still couldn't shift the fear that, deep down, he was a carbon copy of his father, shallow and selfish. And that meant if he had a proper relationship with her, there was a risk he'd end up hurting her.

Plus he knew he didn't have to cheat for things to go wrong between himself and Mandy.

His job was partly in the public eye. He'd seen the kind of things people said about him on social media. That ridiculous nickname of being the thinking woman's crumpet—his team teased him about it, but it was still a real issue. When people saw you on the TV, they formed an opinion about you and they felt that they knew you. And they talked about you. Misinterpreted things. A social kiss on the cheek, an arm round someone's shoulders in a gesture of sympathy, the squeeze of a hand to bolster someone's confidence—it could all be so easily misconstrued.

Sure, these things could be resolved by talking about them.

But it would be like water dripping on a stone. Each tiny droplet of doubt would add to the one before, until eventually it wore away the trust.

And he didn't want that for either of them.

There was only one way he could think of to protect her from that. To protect himself, too. He needed to end things between them. *Now.*

Knowing that this was going to hurt her, but convinced that it would hurt less now than if he let things continue so they got even closer and then it went wrong, he said, 'I like you too, Mandy. Very much.' He steeled himself and added, 'But I'm sorry—I don't want a relationship.'

Shock and hurt flared in her eyes. 'But…we've been getting on so well. I thought that was what you wanted, too.'

'I'm sorry,' he said again. 'I think it's better if we stick to being just colleagues, from now on. I know we're both professional enough not to make things awkward at work.'

For a moment, he thought she was going to argue.

If she did, there was a very good chance he'd fold. Right now, every sinew, every muscle, was screaming out to him to wrap his arms round her and tell her to ignore whatever he'd said because he was panicking and he was being an idiot. Keeping his distance from her felt like physical pain—as if he couldn't breathe. As if he was drowning in fear.

She stared at him for a long, long moment. He saw a muscle flicker in her jaw. Then she said, quietly and tonelessly, 'Then I think I'd better go. I'll see myself out.'

He made no move to stop her when she stood up, slipped her shoes back on and collected her bag and coat from the coat pegs in his hallway. He didn't follow her to the front door, or open it for her.

Only when he heard the door close did he close his eyes and rest his head in his hands.

It was over.

At his own instigation.

And how he wished that things could've been different. That *he* could've been different. That he could've been the right one for her.

But the fear that he wasn't had been too much for him.

CHAPTER ELEVEN

ALL THE WAY HOME, Mandy went over the day in her head. They'd had such a nice time, taking a leisurely stroll round a beautiful hidden garden, enjoying lunch and then browsing in the little shops in Hampstead. They'd laughed, they'd held hands, they'd been close...

And then everything had changed.

Well, she knew what had changed. She'd suggested making their relationship more formal. Going public.

But Daniel had already met her daughter. He'd got on well with Gemma.

He'd introduced her to his sister and brother-in-law, too, and she'd got on well with Ally and Jake.

It worked between them. The last month had been one of the happiest of her life, and he'd seemed happy, too. So why had he backed off? Was it her fault? Had she done something wrong?

She thought about it for the rest of the evening, and still couldn't come up with a convincing reason.

She still hadn't found an answer, the next morning; but at least she could keep herself too busy to think about it by preparing lunch for her mum, her sister and brother-in-law, and Gemma and Dev. And she was super-smiley all afternoon, sidestepping the subject of Daniel when Gemma tried to raise it and instead telling them all about the garden she'd visited with a friend.

They didn't need to know that her 'friend' was now strictly her colleague.

On Monday, she didn't have the usual spring in her step when she walked from the Tube station to the hospital. As she walked down the corridor to the children's department, adrenaline made the ends of her fingers tingle. Facing Daniel was going to be awkward—but it would be even more awkward if other people noticed and started asking questions. She was just going to have to be super-professional about it.

He was already at his desk when she walked into their shared office. 'Good morning, Mandy,' he said, glancing up.

'Good morning, Daniel.' She couldn't think of any small talk to save the situation. She could hardly ask him if he'd had a good weekend, given that he'd called it off between them and the shadows under his eyes looked as deep and dark as hers. What now? Did they talk about the weather? 'I, um—just going to check on a couple of patients,' she said, and fled for the safety of the ward.

Isabella was definitely looking brighter. She still had a slight temperature, but she was smiling and chatty, and her skin wasn't so pallid.

'Look what Dr Dan bought me to say thank you for being in his film!' she said, showing the tutu-wearing mouse to Mandy. 'And, guess what? When he gave it to me, he did a turn just like a ballerina, with his hands up and everything!' She giggled. 'Except he had crabby hands!'

The turn Mandy had taught him, and would've liked to see—except today that might've made her heart crack into pieces. 'That's lovely,' she said, forcing herself to smile broadly. 'Did you tell him they should be flowers?'

'I showed him how and then he did it right,' Isabella confirmed.

'How are you feeling?'

'Ever so much better. Thank you,' she added swiftly at her mum's raised eyebrows. 'Can I go home now, please?'

'In a couple of days,' Mandy said. 'We still need to give you a little bit more medicine.'

Mrs Moran was smiling and looking a lot less

anxious. 'It's going to be hard to keep her in bed, now she's back to her usual self.'

'She can get up and walk about—that's walk, not dance, Bella,' Mandy said. 'Just be careful that she doesn't knock the chest drain or the line where the antibiotics go in. The sputum culture results should be back today, so we'll know if we need to give Bella a different antibiotic, and once the chest drain is out and her temperature's back to normal she can go home.'

'It'll be good to have her home,' Mrs Moran said. 'And thank you for everything you've done, you and Dr Dan.'

You and Dr Dan.

Except they weren't a couple any more. Maybe she'd been kidding herself and they'd never really been one in the first place. She pushed the thought away and made herself smile. 'It's what we're here for.'

Dan loathed himself. He'd seen the shadows under Mandy's eyes, and he knew he'd put them there by breaking up with her. He'd made her miserable.

But what else could he have done?

He focused on running the ward while she was teaching. On Monday evening, he forced himself to ignore how much he missed her and how he wished he was at the cinema with her, or talking to her about all the deep questions over a glass of wine, or lying with her in the bed that suddenly felt much too wide.

Though he missed her.

Really, really missed her.

In the few short weeks they'd been together, he realised that he'd fallen for her. Head over heels. He liked her warmth and her brightness. He liked the way she saw solutions instead of problems. He liked how easy it was to just *be*, in her company.

Right now he was miserable. Nothing in his life seemed to fit, any more, except his job. And that no longer felt like enough.

Mandy was glad that Tuesday was Linda's husband's birthday, so her best friend was taking him out to dinner instead of doing their usual aerobics class. It gave her a couple more days to work out how to avoid Dan's name coming up in conversation.

Wednesday was trickier. She and Dan were scrupulously professional on the handover day. Isabella was going home, the next day, so Dan would be doing a last bit of filming with her; baby Noah was finally able to breathe on his own and was starting to get better; and Joe, despite saying that the liquid nutrition was the most disgusting stuff he'd ever tasted, had responded well and was putting on weight. He was due to start the infliximab, the following week.

But Daniel looked tired, Mandy thought. He wasn't quite as smiley as usual.

Maybe he felt as sad as she did about the way things had gone wrong between them. But his whole 'I don't want a relationship' stance made her wonder if that was the root of the problem. He'd said that he'd forgiven himself for his mistake all those years ago—but had he really? Because he'd struck her as very much a family man, close to his siblings, his nephews and his nieces. The 'book' they'd made him for his fiftieth birthday had been full of love. He would've made a fantastic dad; had he missed out on having children because he didn't trust himself to get it right in his next relationship?

They needed an honest talk.

When he came in to write up his notes, she said, 'Do you want a mug of tea?'

'Thanks, but I'm fine.'

'Are you all right, Dan?' she asked.

'Yes, thank you,' he said coolly.

'You don't look it,' she said. And then, because he was obviously not going to admit to anything unless she said it first, she added, 'You look as miserable as I feel.'

'We're not having this conversation,' Dan said.

'Not here,' she agreed. 'But we do need to talk.'

'We're fine as we are. Colleagues.'

'If you're trying to fake it until you make it, don't. You *know* we're not fine,' she said softly. 'So either we have this conversation here and now, or we go for a drink somewhere quiet after work.'

He didn't say anything, just looked at her. And she was certain she could see a hint of longing in his eyes—that he missed her as much as she missed him. Or was she simply seeing what she so desperately wanted to see?

But then he sighed. 'There's no point, Mandy.'

'No? Then perhaps you can explain this to me. I've seen you working with patients and their parents. I've seen you working with colleagues—from the most junior to the most senior. I've seen you with the film crew. I've seen you with your sister. And the man I see has the most huge heart. He's generous with his time. He's kind. He's thoughtful. But I think he hasn't forgiven himself for a mistake he made nearly thirty years ago. He's shut part of his life off because of that—and I don't understand why.'

'You don't need to understand why,' he said, which told her that she'd been on the right track.

'Oh, but I do,' she said. 'I need to understand why a man who's clearly deeply loved by his nieces and nephews—a man who would've made a wonderful father—denied himself the privilege of having a family of his own.'

He walked over to the open office door and closed it. Then he leaned back against the door. 'All right. If you really want to know, it's because of who I am, deep down. I look like my father—and I behaved like him, too. I cheated and I hurt my wife.'

She blinked, shocked. 'Are you telling me your dad cheated on your mum?'

'Multiple times. I was fifteen when I found out. I asked him why, and he said he'd fallen head over heels for someone else and he couldn't help himself.' Daniel's face tightened. 'But Mum took him back. I thought maybe he'd just made a mistake. Except he did it again. And again. And then I discovered that what I'd thought was the first time was very far from it. He'd cheated all the way through their marriage, and Mum put up with it because she didn't want to drag us all through a divorce.' He dragged in a breath. 'Then, when I fell for Leila…he said I was just like him. It terrified me, because I knew he was right. I'd fallen for someone else when I shouldn't have. And I didn't want to spend the rest of my life being selfish and shallow and un-reliable, not caring if I hurt people—always say-ing sorry and never meaning it, the way he did.'

'But you're not selfish, Dan,' she said. 'Surely you can see that? You're not shallow and un-reliable. You made a mistake and you learned from it.'

'Did I? I can't take the risk,' he said. 'I can't risk hurting you.'

'Does it occur to you that you might be hurt-ing me more by not being in my life?' she asked.

'Yes, and I'm sorry I've hurt you at all, but I can't risk making it worse,' he said. 'I don't trust myself. The apple doesn't fall far from the tree, does it?'

'Your dad might have been a cheat, but your mother wasn't. How do you know you're not more like your mother?' she asked.

'Because if I was, I wouldn't have cheated on Roxy in the first place.'

He was the most stubborn, aggravating man, she thought, circling back to the same argument and not giving himself a chance to break free from all the pain. She tried another tack. 'Don't you think people can change, over time?'

'Some people do. I haven't,' he said. 'Which is why this conversation is going to end now, and we're going back to being strictly colleagues.'

And he flatly refused to discuss the subject with her any more.

It was stalemate. Much as she wanted to yell at him for being stubborn and blinkered, she realised it wouldn't change the situation. Until he was ready to recognise the truth for himself, there was nothing she could do or say to change his mind. And maybe he was so stuck in his ways, after all these years, that he'd never let himself recognise the truth.

So she avoided him as much as she could without making it obvious, told Gemma and Linda quietly that things between her and Dan had simply fizzled out and there wasn't any point in discussing it, and concentrated on her job.

Over the next week, Mandy's cool, professional distance was hard to bear. Daniel *missed* her. He missed the lightness of spirit he'd felt when they were together. He missed her sense of humour.

But he'd been the one to call a halt. He'd been the one to push her away. He knew he only had himself to blame.

On Tuesday morning, he was dealing with a pile of admin when the phone he shared with Mandy shrilled; he picked it up and answered absently. 'Daniel Monroe.'

'Could I speak to Dr Cooke, please?' a voice asked.

'I'm sorry, she's with a patient,' Daniel said. 'Can I help at all? I work with her.'

'Could you get a very urgent message to her, please? It's Dev, her son-in-law,' the voice on the other end of the phone said. 'I'm on my way to the hospital now. Gemma's being brought in by an ambulance. I know she'll want her mum.'

'Of course I will.' Daniel did some rapid calculations in his head. Gemma must be thirty-six weeks pregnant. A month before her due date. That wasn't good. 'Sorry to ask, but can I give Mandy any idea what's happened, so I can prepare her a bit?' he asked.

'Gemma had a bit of a headache this morning, but she still went into work. At the end of the first lesson, she was sick, having stomach pains and her hands were swollen. The school secretary called an ambulance. The paramedics weren't happy with her blood pressure so they're bringing her to hospital.'

'OK,' Daniel said. It had been years since his rotation in the maternity department, but he recognised the symptoms of pre-eclampsia. If it was severe, the only cure was to deliver the baby. Four weeks early wasn't as tough as it could be, but it was still worrying. And there was still the chance that before delivery the pre-eclampsia could progress to full-blown eclampsia. 'I'll go and find her now,' he said. 'Dev, try not to worry. They might need to deliver the baby early, but they're really used to dealing with babies born a bit early, and thirty-six weeks isn't super-early.'

'Uh-huh.' Dev was clearly worried sick but trying to stay calm.

'I'll go and find Mandy now,' he said. 'Can I take your number in case she needs me to pass on a message?'

Dev dictated his number and Daniel read it back to check he'd taken it down correctly. 'Try not to worry,' he said again. 'And call again if you need to.'

He called down to the Emergency Department to see if Gemma was there yet; she wasn't, so he checked the board and discovered that Mandy was in consulting room two. He knocked on the door and stepped inside the doorway. 'Dr Cooke, I'm so sorry to interrupt, but I need an urgent word, please.'

She frowned, but apologised to her patient, their parents and her student for the interruption. 'What is it?' she asked when she'd followed him out of the room.

'I don't want you to worry,' he said, 'but Dev just called.'

'Dev?' Her face blanched. 'What's happened to Gemma?' Her eyes widened with fear. 'If she was too ill to call me herself...'

'She started vomiting at work,' he said, 'and she's got a headache and stomach pains. The paramedics weren't happy with her blood pressure. She's on the way in, and so is Dev, but I think she's going to need her mum.'

Mandy was shaking. 'Oh, God. That sounds like pre-eclampsia.' She didn't say it, but he could see in her expression what was worrying her: *what if it progresses?* 'What was her blood pressure reading?'

'Dev didn't say. But if it's not super-high they might manage her conservatively on the ward.'

'Or they might deliver the baby early.' Mandy bit her lip. 'She's thirty-six weeks. But she never gets headaches. Are her hands and feet swollen? And—'

'We're not going to know any more until the ambulance gets here,' he cut in gently. 'I rang down to the Emergency Department, and she's not here yet. Go now, and Dev's on his way in as well. I'll sort out your patient and your students.'

'But—'

'We're still a team on the ward,' he said softly. 'Gemma needs you. I'll cover for you, and I'll explain to everyone that you're dealing with a family emergency. Call me if you need anything. Otherwise I'll presume you're all be on the maternity ward and I'll check in with you at the end of my shift.'

'Thank you.'

He took her hand and squeezed it. 'Gemma's going to be in the right place if anything happens. Try not to worry.'

Mandy got to the Emergency Department about five minutes after Gemma did.

'Mum.' Her daughter was pale and shaking. 'I...'

'I know, darling, and it's going to be all right,' Mandy soothed, holding her free hand tightly. 'You're in the right place. We'll get this sorted out.' And at least she knew the doctor who was assessing Gemma, having worked with him on a couple of her patients. 'I'm not going to get in the way, Alan,' she reassured him.

'I know,' the younger doctor said, smiling. 'Your mum's one of the good ones, Gemma.'

It was scary to see her daughter with a cannula in her hand to give intravenous access and a monitor on her finger to measure her pulse and blood oxygen saturation, even though she knew they were the first procedures the Emergency Department staff would do.

The next few minutes were a blur while Alan examined Gemma, took bloods and a temperature reading, then a manual blood pressure reading, had a quick conversation with one of the obstetricians and then gave Gemma medication for her blood pressure.

'We're going to transfer you upstairs to Maternity, Gemma, and they'll catheterise you there—we need a wee sample now, and then in Maternity they'll monitor your fluid input and output,' Alan said. 'If your husband checks in at Reception, they'll tell him where to find you. And you've got your mum here to keep an eye on you, too.'

'But you're meant to be at work, Mum,' Gemma said.

'It's fine,' Mandy reassured her. 'Daniel's looking after my students and clinics for me, and I'll sort some of his paperwork in return. I'll message him so he knows what's happening.'

By the time they were in the maternity unit—and Mandy had reassured her daughter that being in the high-dependency section of the ward simply meant the team could keep a really close eye on her, plus it would be quieter than the main ward—Dev had arrived.

'We'll try to get your blood pressure down, Gemma,' Connie, the midwife, said. 'The consultant and the anaesthetist both know you're here, and we'll be keeping regular checks on your blood pressure and your pulse, as well as regular checks on the baby.'

'What's made me ill?' Gemma asked.

'We think you have pre-eclampsia,' Connie said. 'Your mum will be able to tell you about that.'

Mandy smiled. 'It's been a while since I did my maternity rotation. You're more up to date than I am—plus *you're* her midwife. I'm simply here as Gemma's mum.'

Connie gave her a smile of understanding and turned to Gemma. 'It's a complication of pregnancy where your blood pressure's too high and protein leaks from your kidneys into your urine. And sometimes it can affect how your blood clots.'

'What causes it?' Dev asked.

'It's not fully understood, but we know it's a problem with the blood vessels that supply the placenta. It's nothing you've done wrong,' Connie said. 'It's most common in the third trimester, and it's usually picked up at a routine antenatal. Up to six per cent of first pregnancies are affected by it. Some people don't have any symptoms at all; but a headache that just won't go away is a common one, along with being sick, having a pain under your ribs and having swollen hands and feet.'

'How does it affect the baby?' Gemma asked.

'It affects how well the placenta works and the baby's growth,' Connie explained. 'We're keeping an eye on the baby to make sure they're not in distress; you'll have an ultrasound shortly to check the blood flow through the placenta, measure the baby's growth and see how much amniotic fluid there is. We're also going to monitor the baby's heart rate. If we can keep you going with medication and monitoring until thirty-seven weeks and the baby's not in distress, that's when we'll advise you to have the baby—either by induction or by a caesarean section.'

'What if the baby's in distress?' Dev asked.

'Then we'll suggest delivering the baby now,' Connie said. 'You're at thirty-six weeks, so the baby will be only a tiny bit premature. If it makes you feel any better, we often deliver twins at thirty-five weeks. Try not to worry.'

Gemma looked relieved.

'We'll need to keep you in a little bit longer than usual after delivery, to make sure there aren't any complications, and your little one might need a short stay in the neonatal unit so we can keep a close eye on them, but try not to worry. The main thing is we'll keep an eye on you both and keep you safe. And your midwife and health visitor will check your blood pressure more regularly until it's back to normal and you stop needing the medication.'

'Will I get it again if we have another baby?' Gemma asked.

'It's possible, but because we know it happened in your first pregnancy we can monitor you more closely in any future pregnancies,' Connie said.

The rest of the morning felt like an endless round of tests and discussions, though Mandy was pleased to see that the maternity team took the same approach as the children's ward, making sure their patients understood the choices.

Finally the consultant said, 'I'm not happy with your blood pressure, Gemma. Obviously it's your choice, but I'd like to deliver the baby.'

'Will I at least be awake for it?' Gemma asked.

'Yes. We can give you spinal anaesthesia,' he said. 'And Dev can be in there with you to hold your hand.'

'Then I'll pop back to my ward for a few minutes,' Mandy said. 'Everything's going to be fine, Gemma. I'll see you very soon.' She kissed her daughter and her son-in-law, then headed back to the ward.

Daniel was in their joint office. 'How's Gemma?' he asked.

'She has pre-eclampsia,' Mandy said. 'Her blood pressure's been a bit stubborn, so she's having a section now.' She bit her lip. 'This is when being a doctor isn't so great. You know all the complications.'

'And you also know the solutions,' he reminded her. 'She's in the right place.'

'I know. But it's my job to worry about her,' Mandy said. 'Thank you for covering my clinics this morning—and the first half of this afternoon.'

'Not a problem,' he said. 'I had a couple of meetings that were easily moved. It's all fine. I assume you're going back to Maternity now?'

'I ought to finish my clinic, first,' she said.

'Go back to Gemma,' he said. 'I'll handle your clinic. You'd do the same for me, if I were in your shoes.'

'True,' she admitted.

'Go. And I'll come and see you at the end of the shift and fill you in.' He smiled. 'And sneak a cuddle. There's nothing like newborn cuddles.'

'Thank you. I really appreciate your support,' Mandy said.

It was the least he could do, Daniel thought, but he didn't say it.

At the end of his shift, he went up to see Gemma and Dev. He found them by their newborn's crib in the neonatal unit; Gemma was in a wheelchair.

'Thank you for everything you did for us today, Daniel,' Gemma said. 'Sorry I can't stand up to greet you properly. It'll be another couple of hours before the spinal block's worn off.'

Dev shook his hand warmly. 'Thank you for getting Mandy to be with Gemma so quickly.'

'You're very welcome,' Daniel said with a smile. 'And your baby's beautiful.'

'He needs a little bit of special care right now,' Gemma said, 'but we're hoping in a day or two he can join me in my room.'

'They'll want to keep an eye on his breathing, temperature and blood sugar, and catch any jaundice early,' Daniel said. 'Though you should be able to feed him yourself, if that's what you'd planned. The neonatal team will teach you and Dev things like kangaroo care—where you hold him against your chest, skin to skin—and "comfort holding". And they're very used to questions, so feel free to ask them anything.'

'I feel a bit daft, asking if a thirty-six-week-old baby counts as premature,' she said, wrinkling her nose.

She had Mandy's lovely brown eyes, and it made him feel warm inside. 'Thirty-six weeks officially counts as late preterm,' Daniel said, 'but remember that full term is anything from thirty-seven weeks. So he might be in the unit for a few days, but during that time his care will transition to you.' He paused. 'Where's your mum?'

'She's gone to pick up my hospital bag,' Gemma said. 'Actually, I could do with a drink of water.

Would you mind pushing me back to my room while Dev stays with the baby, please?'

Daniel was pretty sure there was a water cooler in the unit, but clearly Gemma wanted to talk to him about something in private. 'Sure,' he said.

She waited until they were back in her room. 'I don't know what went wrong between you and Mum,' she said gently, 'but I wish it hadn't. She was happier with you than she'd been in a long time.'

He winced. 'It's complicated.'

'Does it have to be?' she asked. 'When I saw you together, it was pretty clear that you were in love with each other. I know Mum can be a bit guarded sometimes, but she's special.'

'She deserves someone who'll treat her properly,' he said.

'She does,' Gemma agreed. 'And I thought that someone was you.'

'I'm the worst person she could get involved with,' Daniel said. 'My marriage broke up because I was unfaithful.'

'Obviously you must know my dad cheated on her, if infidelity's the reason why you think you're wrong for her,' Gemma said. 'Can I be rude and ask, did it happen very long ago?'

'I was about your age,' he admitted.

She raised her eyebrows. 'That's a whole generation ago. And you've really not forgiven yourself in all that time? I think you've been too hard on yourself, Dan. Everyone makes mistakes. Sometimes really terrible ones. But that doesn't mean you should just give up. So learn from whatever you did and move on.'

He couldn't. He was stuck. So he just stared at her.

'I can't remember the last time my mum dated someone. But she trusted you enough to let you close,' Gemma said thoughtfully. 'And—my dad aside, obviously—she's a good judge of character. If Mum can trust you, maybe you should follow her lead and trust yourself.'

'Maybe,' he said, not wanting to argue with her. 'Let me get you that glass of water and push you back to join your husband and son.'

Just as he'd handed Gemma the water, Mandy walked in.

'I've got the hospital bag for you,' she said.

'Thanks, Mum.' Gemma gave her a grateful smile.

'Your grandson is gorgeous,' Daniel said. 'I'm not going to ask for a cuddle now, because I know he's more vulnerable to infections and he needs to rest—which doesn't happen when he's being passed round to people. But I'm definitely claiming a cuddle when he's ready to socialise.'

'You've got it,' Gemma said. 'Can we go back, now?'

'Sure.' He wheeled her back to the neonatal unit.

'Mum, you need a break. You've been watching over me or running errands all day,' Gemma said.

'So unsubtle, Gem,' Dev said with a sigh. 'You're supposed to point out that our baby can only have two visitors at a time, and right now that's you and me, and my parents are on their way down from Manchester and will be here any minute now, so maybe we can catch up with your mum tomorrow?'

'Very tactful, Dev,' Gemma said.

'We get the message. We'll leave you in peace,' Mandy said.

At the door to the neonatal unit, she said to Daniel, 'You've clearly been looking after Gemma in my absence. Thank you.'

'You're very welcome. She's lovely.'

And her words echoed in his head. *If Mum can trust you, maybe you should follow her lead and trust yourself...*'

Could he try?

'Mandy.'

'Yes?'

'You've had a day of worrying yourself sick,' he said. 'Come home with me. I'll feed you and drive you home.'

'I don't think that's a good idea,' she said.

'And I'd like to talk,' he added softly. 'I know I haven't been fair to you. I understand if you don't want to go to my place. Maybe we can just find somewhere quiet in King's Cross where we can grab something to eat and have the space to talk? Neutral territory.'

For a very long and very nasty moment, he thought she might refuse.

But then she huffed out a breath. 'I'm too tired and too stressed to cook tonight,' she admitted.

'No strings,' he said. 'Something to eat, and a quiet chat.'

'All right.'

They didn't speak much on the way to King's Cross, but it wasn't an awkward silence so he didn't mind.

'Fancy some comfort food?' he asked.

'I'm thinking macaroni cheese,' she said.

'Good call.'

They found a café offering what they wanted, and ordered two big bowls of macaroni cheese with a dish of steamed tenderstem broccoli cooked with garlic and lemon. Daniel added a jug of water and two glasses of prosecco to their order.

'Prosecco? Seriously?'

'We're both too tired to drink a whole bottle between us, and we need to toast the baby,' he said.

She gave him a weary smile. 'We do. That was scary, today. I didn't tell Gemma, obviously, but in my head I was running through the stats of how frequently pre-eclampsia turns to eclampsia.'

Just what he'd guessed. 'One less worry is that he's thirty-six weeks,' Daniel said, 'so he didn't need steroids to help mature his lungs.'

'But there's the risk of jaundice.'

'Which is easily fixed with phototherapy,' he countered.

'True.' She closed her eyes. 'That's the thing about your children. When you see them upset and worried and ill, you want to take it all from them so everything's OK again. You'd do anything to have a real magic wand.'

'That goes for nieces and nephews, too,' Daniel said. 'At least for me, as they're the closest I have to children.'

She opened her eyes again. 'You would've made a good dad.'

'I made a different choice,' he said. But maybe, just maybe, he could be a grandad…

Though that was running before he could walk. He needed to be totally honest with Mandy before he could even think about suggesting something like that. Take the risk and really open his heart to her.

He was about to open his mouth and tell her when the waiter came up with their prosecco.

So instead he smiled. 'To Gemma, Dev and the baby,' he said, lifting his glass.

'Gemma, Dev and the baby,' she echoed.

They lapsed into silence again when their food arrived. She picked at her meal, he noticed. 'Sorry,' she said. 'The food's good. I think I'm just too tired to eat.'

'It sounds as if you've hit that point when you know you can stop worrying quite so much, and at the same time you realise just how much you *have* been worrying and it wipes you out,' he said. 'I've been there.' He pushed his own plate away and looked at her. 'Gemma said something that made me think. If you can trust me not to cheat on you, maybe I should follow your lead and trust myself.'

'Gemma said that?' Her eyes widened. 'I didn't tell her anything about what you told me in confidence.'

'I know. I told her about it myself,' he said. 'But she didn't judge me. She asked me how old I was at the time, and pointed out that it happened a whole generation ago.'

Mandy laced her fingers together, resting her

elbows on the table and her chin on her linked fingers. 'Did you listen to her?'

'I should,' he said, 'have listened to *you* when you said something very like it in the first place.' He sighed. 'The idea of a proper relationship terrifies me. I was desperate to make a go of my marriage with Roxy, prove to myself that I wasn't my dad. And what happened? I did exactly what my dad would've done.'

'Maybe,' she said, 'you rushed into marriage. You met Roxy when you were both eighteen, and people change hugely between that age and twenty-five.'

'I know,' he said softly. 'I thought we'd change together. But we grew apart, instead. I don't think either of us knew how tough those years would be, with me working stupid hours and studying and not spending enough time with her. I wouldn't have blamed her for leaving me for someone else—someone who was prepared to put the work into their relationship. For me, that made it even worse that I was the one who looked elsewhere, not her.'

'So you've punished yourself ever since, convinced that you're shallow and unreliable,' she said. 'When you're not. The truth is, you were both young and you found yourselves in a situation neither of you really had the tools to cope with at the time.' She paused. 'You said Roxy forgave you.'

'She did.'

'So follow her lead,' she said. 'Forgive yourself.'

'The thing is, I've thought of myself in those terms for so long, I don't even know where to start,' he said.

'People are capable of changing, if they really want to,' she said gently. 'It sounds to me as if your dad didn't want to change; he was quite happy putting himself first. Whereas you—you don't do that.'

'Don't I?'

'No. Would your father have taken Daisy for a walk by the sea and told her she didn't have to be a doctor, then made her think about doing something that combined the caring side of medicine with the music and dance she loved so much?' she asked.

'Well, no. He would have seen her as the third generation of medics in our family. And he probably would've tried to pressure her into following in his exact footsteps and becoming a surgeon,' Daniel said.

'Exactly. Putting himself first. Not like you. And you're the same at work. You put yourself in other people's shoes. You thought how I'd react to the news about Gemma coming into hospital, and knew that I'd want to be with her—so you told me to be with her while you sorted everything else out.' She looked at him. 'And I knew I'd be safe to leave my patients and my students in your hands, because you're reliable.'

'Even though I let you down?'

'You've spent so long thinking about yourself as the bad guy, you've forgotten to remember the good stuff you do,' she said. 'You learned how to do a ballet turn, just to make a little girl smile.'

'She was so pleased,' he said. 'And you were right. She told me I was holding my fingers wrong. She said they were crabby and they should be flowers.' He smiled. 'It was good to see her giggle, given how pale and poorly she was when she came in.'

'That's why I didn't tell you how to hold your hands,' Mandy said. 'I thought she'd enjoy teaching you.'

'She did.'

'And there's Matty. I bet you end up going to watch him play cricket.'

'Busted,' Daniel muttered. 'I was planning to do that in the summer.'

'So are you going to start trying to see your good side?' she asked.

'I want to. I really want to,' he said. 'But I think I'm going to need help.'

'You told our team that asking for help when

you need it is a sign of strength,' Mandy said. 'Maybe you should take your own advice.'

Hope flooded through him. If she meant that… 'Will you give me a second chance, Mandy?' he asked. 'And help me learn to give myself a second chance?' He shook his head. 'No, that's coming out all wrong. It's all me, me, me, and that's not what I want.'

'What do you want?' she asked.

'Love,' he said simply. 'I love you, Mandy. I think I fell for you the first day I met you, when you told me terrible—and literally—cheesy jokes. You make my world a brighter place, and I want to do that for you, too. I want to share my life with you. Explore things with you, to learn and laugh and…love,' he finished.

'That's what I want, too,' she said. 'But that means opening up to me. Trusting me, and trusting yourself. Can you do that?'

'With you by my side, yes. I'm always going to worry,' he admitted, 'but knowing that you believe in me will help to stem the doubts.'

'You're a good man, Daniel Monroe,' she said. 'I love you. Let's see if we can change the way you think about you.' She reached over to take his hand. 'Starting now.'

EPILOGUE

Three months later

ON AN UNUSUALLY sunny Saturday morning in late February, Mandy walked hand in hand with Daniel through the grounds of the gorgeous seventeenth-century Ham House.

'That's an amazing house,' she said. 'I bet the gardens are full of roses in the summer.'

'We'll come back and find out, but I wanted to come this weekend because I had something specific in mind,' Daniel said. And suddenly he felt ridiculously nervous. What if…?

But Mandy had taught him to believe in himself over the last three months. And his world had really opened up. Everything from hosting family lunches where everyone brought a dish to add to the kitchen table already groaning with what he'd cooked, through to baby James Devendra Shastri's christening, the previous week—where he'd been incredibly touched and proud that Gemma and Dev had asked him to be one of the baby's godfathers.

He encouraged Mandy to keep up with her book group, dance aerobics and ballet class, just as she encouraged him to keep up going to the gym with his best friend; and he and Mandy had a regular Wednesday night slot babysitting James to give Gemma and Dev a chance of spending time together. He'd loved bathtime, lullabies and storytime; being an unofficial step-grandparent had really enriched his life.

And in between, he got to wake up with Mandy in his arms every morning—either at his place or hers—and to spend time with the loveliest woman he'd ever met.

She nudged him.

'What?' he asked.

'You were away with the fairies. What's this specific thing? Have you been reading guide-books again?'

'Websites,' he said. And the picture he'd found had made him realise this was going to be the perfect backdrop for what he had in mind. He'd checked with Gemma first, on the quiet, and she'd given him the most enormous hug, followed by asking a question that had actually brought tears to his eyes and a lump to his throat.

'And...?' Mandy prompted.

'There was something I wanted you to see in the gardens,' he said.

'Snowdrops?' she asked. 'I love snowdrops.'

'There are snowdrops,' he said, 'but that's not it.' As they walked through the grounds towards the back of the house, he said, 'Would you humour me and close your eyes until I say you can open them?'

She laughed. 'I don't have a clue why you're asking that, but all right. I trust you not to let me walk straight through a puddle or fall flat on my face.'

He led her along the gravelled path until they reached the back of the house—and the photo he'd seen from the previous spring that had caught his eye barely did it justice.

'All right,' he said, drawing them both to a halt in front of one of the large rectangular areas. 'You can open your eyes now.'

She did so. 'That's gorgeous! A purple carpet—of crocuses? I've never seen anything like this. My favourite colour, too.'

He knew. It was why he'd chosen this spot.

She grinned. 'No wonder you sounded so pleased with yourself when you asked me to close my eyes.'

'I wanted the perfect backdrop.' He went down on one knee. 'Amanda Cooke, I think I fell in

love with you the first day I met you—and it's
not just cupboard love because you make the best
brownies. You've changed my life for the better,
and you've taught me to do something I haven't
done for half a lifetime: to trust myself. I asked
Gemma's permission, and she said I could ask
you.' The words spilled out in a rush. 'Will you
marry me?'

Her smile broadened and she opened her arms
to welcome him. 'I love you, too, Dan. Yes.'

He stood up, wrapped his arms round her, and
kissed her until he was dizzy. 'Thank you,' he
said. 'I haven't bought a ring, because I thought
it'd be nice to choose it together. Maybe we can
go shopping this afternoon.'

'I'd like that,' she said. 'But backtrack a moment. You asked my daughter's permission?'

'She was really pleased that I'd asked.' He
swallowed the lump in his throat. 'And she asked
if she could call me "Dad".'

'Oh!' Mandy's eyes filmed with tears, telling
him that she was affected in the same way that
he'd been.

'Shall we give her the answer?' he asked,
taking his phone from his pocket and flicking
into the camera app. They stood with their arms
wrapped round each other, smiling, and he an-

gled the screen so the carpet of purple crocuses was the full background.

And then he sent the picture to Gemma.

The answer's yes. To both questions. xx

* * * * *

*If you enjoyed this story,
check out these other great reads from
Kate Hardy*

Sparks Fly with the Single Dad
An English Vet in Paris
Saving Christmas for the ER Doc
Surgeon's Second Chance in Florence

All available now!

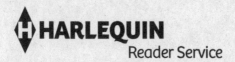
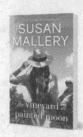
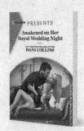
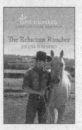
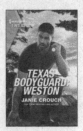